EP Sport Series

Tennis up to Tournament
Standard

Modern Riding

Sailing

Table Tennis

Learning to Swim

Snooker

Squash Rackets

EP PUBLISHING LIMITED 1975

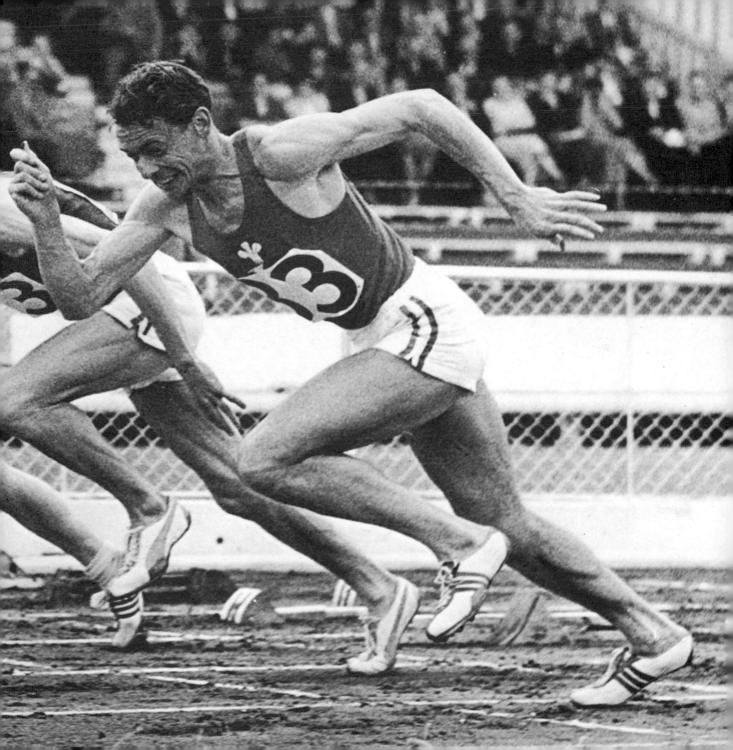

conditioning
for sport

dr. n. whitehead
principal lecturer,
carnegie school of
physical education, leeds

The author

The author would like to
acknowledge with thanks the
assistance of the following in the
preparation of the book:

John Dodd, Gordon, and Yorkshire
TV for various photographs.

Colleagues, students and friends for
posing for the photographs.

ISBN 0 7158 0593 2

Published by EP Publishing Ltd, East Ardsley,
Wakefield, West Yorkshire, 1975

Text set in 11/12 pt. Photon Univers, printed by
photolithography, and bound in Great Britain at
The Pitman Press, Bath.

Contents

Introduction

Progress

Undoubtedly there has been progress in recent years in the standards of performance of various sportsmen and sportswomen. One of the major factors that has enabled this progress to take place is the advance in the knowledge of what happens to the body when we participate in sport, and how the body can be conditioned to play harder, move faster and withstand a greater volume of work before fatigue sets in.

Older people might claim that sportsmen in the past were as good as those of the present. They might say that Joe Louis was as good a heavyweight as Muhammad Ali, that Stanley Matthews was as good a soccer player as Georgie Best, and that Maureen Connolly was as good a tennis player as Billie-Jean King. But if we turn to sports in which present-day standards can be *measured* against those of the past, then we can observe that Johnny Weissmuller's Olympic swimming performance would be beaten by most international *women* swimmers these days, and the great Paavo Nurmi's long distance running times are nowadays attainable by schoolboys. Therefore it could be justifiably claimed that today's sports stars are generally *fitter* than those of the past.

Variety in Training

Earlier this century, training (if carried out at all) consisted mainly of practising the sports or skills involved in the particular game. If a keen sportsman decided to do anything extra it would take the form of either a short cross-country run or a few laps of a games field. There were a number of reasons for this, including the belief that too much effort strained the heart, a fear that a person could become "muscle-bound", the necessity of avoiding "staleness" and the misapprehension that training practices were only valuable if related to the actual skills performed in the game. Modern coaches believe that a wide variety of conditioning routines not only ensures a more balanced physiological development of sportsmen and sportswomen, but also helps to ward off boredom.

Different Sports— Different Conditioning

The new knowledge acquired for instance on strength training and endurance work has reached a high level of sophistication. Not only are most sportsmen recommended to lift weights (unheard-of twenty years ago in most sports), they are also urged to do a large quantity of sprinting in lieu of the formerly used cross-country runs. Furthermore, **individual** fitness schedules are recommended, and can be designed for **every single** sportsman whether he plays in a team game or not.

This is the purpose of this book—to outline the components of different sports, and to provide a guide for coaches who wish to plan schedules of conditioning or "fitness training" for the sportsmen and women in their care.

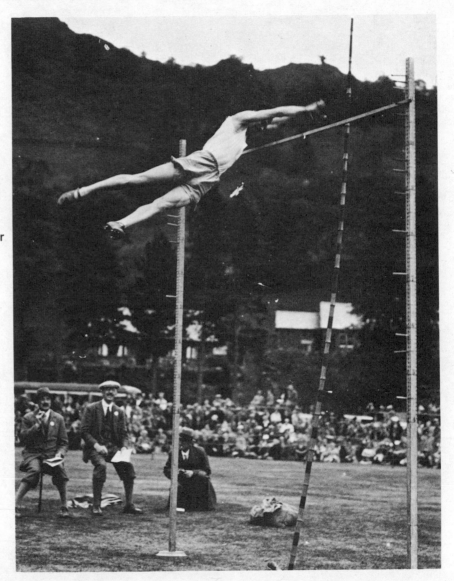

A competitor winning a pole vault competition in the English Lake District in 1934 at a height 6 inches *higher* than the winning vault in 1974!
Note a spiked bamboo pole was used, and there was no soft landing bed.

Principles of Conditioning

Fitness

"A person physically fit in all respects does not exist."

Karpovich, 1965

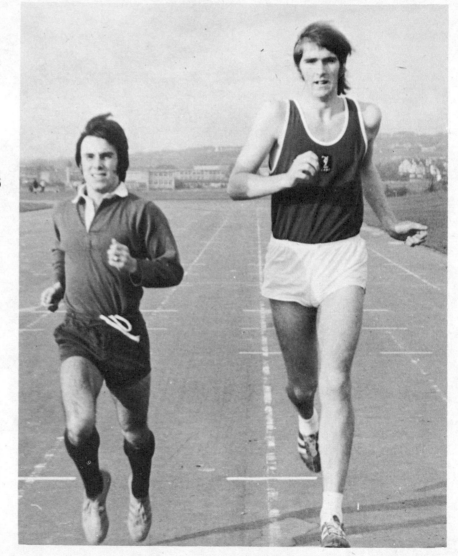

Both of these sportsmen would claim to be "very fit". But the one on the left is a top class hockey player, the one on the right a top-class basketball player. If they were required to participate in a sport other than their own, they would realise that they are not as "fit" as they thought!

Despite the progress made in various games and sports in recent years, one of the most astonishing features that results from discussion with many top class coaches is the lack of agreement on the subject of "fitness". Very many coaches and sports stars use the term in a fashion which often gives the impression that they really do not know a great deal about the subject. Many refer to "fitness" as though it is a condition to be found in an identical fashion in swimmers, footballers or other performers. The fact is that a person who is "fit" for swimming could be completely "unfit" for football, and a "fit" track and field athlete could be "unfit" by gymnastic standards. Furthermore, though coaches would accept that a "fit" sprinter should not necessarily be expected to be as "fit" to run 10,000 metres as a "fit" 10,000 metres runner, the same coaches do not always accept that within particular games, a "fit" defender in

football could well be "unfit" for duties in attack in the same game. This is illustrated by the fact that some football coaches give all of their players the same "fitness" training work regardless of the position in which the player normally participates.

This book attempts to impress upon the reader that "getting fit" for a sport is a process that will differ for **every individual** whether he plays in team games or individual sports. The process consists of getting a number of systems in an individual's body into the **appropriate condition** relative to the requirements of a good performance in his own sporting activity.

However, when ascertaining which are the best methods to acquire the appropriate conditions within the body for a number of men and women and a number of different sports, some similarities will be seen to exist. Most sportsmen move about during their activities,

therefore **running** would often seem to be a common component. Most sports necessitate performance over a long period of time, therefore an **endurance** factor would seem to be common. Other requisites would appear to be varying degrees of **strength** and **flexibility** in the musculature and joints, as well as the **skills** required in the sport and the correct psychological preparation for the performance of those skills.

This chapter of the book deals with these components of "fitness" or "conditioning", and it is hoped that it will enable sportsmen and coaches to understand why "fitness training" or "conditioning" must be specific for each individual, and **not** simply a mass of exercises or practices provided for a variety of sportsmen, to be performed by all at the same time, using the same amount of effort.

Frequently, one hears of references to "stamina" in discussions on training. Though the author is not an advocate of using vague terminology when simple English will suffice, it is considered that it is unhelpful to use the old term of "stamina" work which is associated with old practices of cross-country runs, or the running of laps around games fields. A more accurate picture is obtained if one thinks of "stamina" as being subdivided into two forms:

(a) circulo-respiratory endurance, and

(b) muscular endurance.

Circulo-Respiratory Endurance

". . . a measure of an efficient heart and lung system."

Pickering, 1968

In simple terms, this describes the ability of the circulatory system (heart and blood supply) and the respiratory system (lungs and breathing) to withstand periods of hard work.
It is essential for coaches and sportsmen to know a small amount of what is happening within the body during exercise so that programmes of training can be planned more realistically. The minimum of such information could be summarised as follows.
The energy that is stored in muscles consists of glycogen (which includes oxygen), protein, fat etc.

During exercise, the muscle action results in the glycogen being used up and it is replaced by lactic acid. The longer the exercise continues, the greater the build-up of lactic acid and the diminishing of oxygen, and the more the muscles become fatigued (this is called an "oxygen debt"). The way to overcome this fatigue is by ensuring that the heart and lungs are improved in efficiency so that they can pump more oxygen to the working muscles, because the presence of oxygen removes the lactic acid. But the conditioning of the circulo-respiratory system aims not only to produce more oxygen to convert the lactic acid, but also to train the body to tolerate the lactic acid and the feeling of fatigue until the oxygen supply arrives. That is, rather than urging sportsmen to take rests when they feel fatigued, so that the body can have time to replace the lactic acid with oxygen, coaches should **expect** sportsmen to become breathless during training

These are two of Britain's leading middle distance men. To the layman or to a person from another sport, they may simply appear to be thin, bony young men, whereas in fact they represent the epitome of circulo-respiratory endurance.

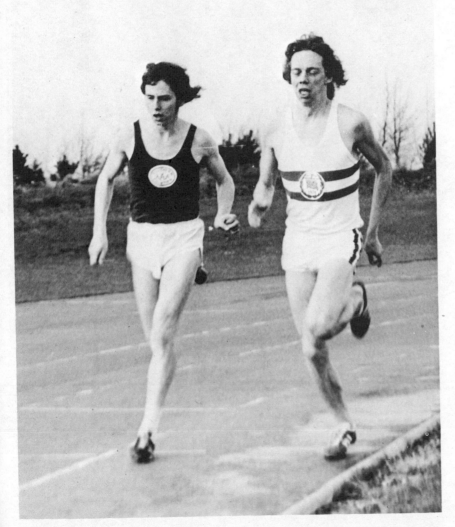

sessions as indeed they will during competition.

To condition the body for this "oxygen debt", or build-up of lactic acid, or simple fatigue, a number of programmes can be devised and these are described in a later chapter, but it is appropriate to emphasise here that there are methods other than long-distance runs that will achieve the correct effect.

Muscular Endurance

"... The capacity of a group of
muscles to continue working
withstanding fatigue as long as
possible."

Pickering, 1968

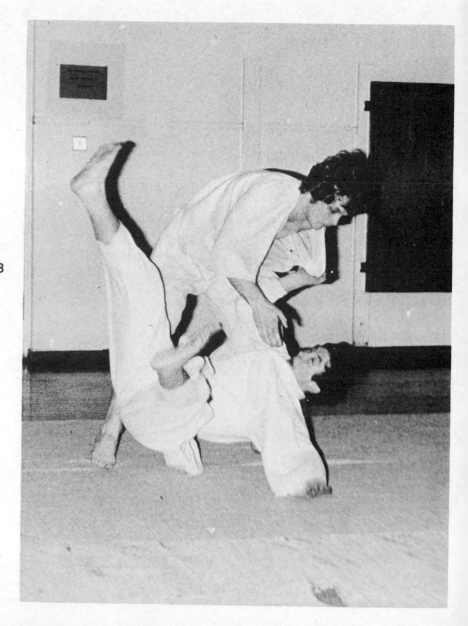

Muscular endurance is to be found in
greatest amounts in such sports as judo,
wrestling, and boxing where the
emphasis is on non-stop activity of the
whole body.

16

This is another form of "stamina" often unknown to or misunderstood by coaches. Whereas it is a generally recognised need in training sessions to ensure that sportsmen become breathless (circulo-respiratory endurance), often no attempt is made to ensure that in the muscle groups essential to particular sportsmen, a "jelly-like" feeling of fatigue is obtained, that is a **local** endurance as opposed to an **overall** feeling of exhaustion. Though an individual's muscular endurance is closely linked to the efficiency of his circulo-respiratory endurance, the best illustration of the need to do specific training in the former is the action of sawing a piece of wood. A good long-distance runner will have a good degree of circulo-respiratory endurance, but this will not enable him to saw wood more efficiently than a person who is not so good a runner. In fact, if this not-so-good runner uses his arms daily in activities such as blacksmith work, carpentry, or sweeping the streets, *he* is more likely to be better at sawing wood. That is to say, both types of endurance work are essential in differing degrees, depending upon the sport and the particular duties of the sportsman.

Specifically, muscular endurance training ensures a more efficient circulation of the blood through the muscles, so a greater amount of "energy" is stored within the muscles, and this "energy" is more readily available in the muscles during exercise.

Strength

"...The ability of the muscle to exert force against resistance."

Adamson, 1961

Much confusion also exists in the minds of coaches and sportsmen relating to the concept of "strength". Many attempt to show their understanding by using such terminology as "dynamic strength", "static strength", "power", "force", etc. But there would appear to be little need to go beyond the use of the word "strength" providing the person involved realises that strengthening implies a process enabling a person to, say, lift heavier weights than he was able to lift before. Many present-day "strengthening" programmes give weight-training schedules for sportsmen to lift that enable the sportsmen to **lift the same weight** more times as the weeks progress, but not necessarily heavier weights. That is to say, many so-called "strength" sessions are in fact "muscular-endurance" sessions. The simple difference physiologically between muscular-endurance work and strengthening is that in the former, a greater efficiency is aimed for in the blood supply to the muscles, whereas in **strength** work we are aiming to increase the size of the muscles, and the number of muscle fibres to be used during the sporting activity. Improved strength enables a sportsman to apply more force in an activity because of the improved size and condition of the **muscle fibres,** and not (as in the case of muscular endurance) mainly the blood supply to the muscles. This could be illustrated by saying that strength work enables a footballer to kick a ball further, whereas muscular endurance work would enable him to continue kicking a ball for a long period of time.

At this juncture, it is appropriate to stress that planned strengthening work does **not** result in sportsmen becoming "muscle-bound", neither are carefully selected strengthening programmes harmful to women. It is probably true to say that as many injuries occur in strength training as in other types of training, but these are more often due to bad instruction in the techniques of performing the exercises than the nature of the exercises. A further point to be made is to debunk the fallacy that strength work slows down a sportsman. Added strength will enable an individual to cover ground faster, strike an object harder and further, and generally enable the person to play a better game or perform an activity at an improved standard.

Strength is essential to the top class
rugby prop forward in this photograph,
for his role is not only to push in the set
scrummages, but to attempt to barge
his way through situations such as illustrated. However for part of the game
he is also required to run around the
field, therefore he cannot depend solely
upon strength training.

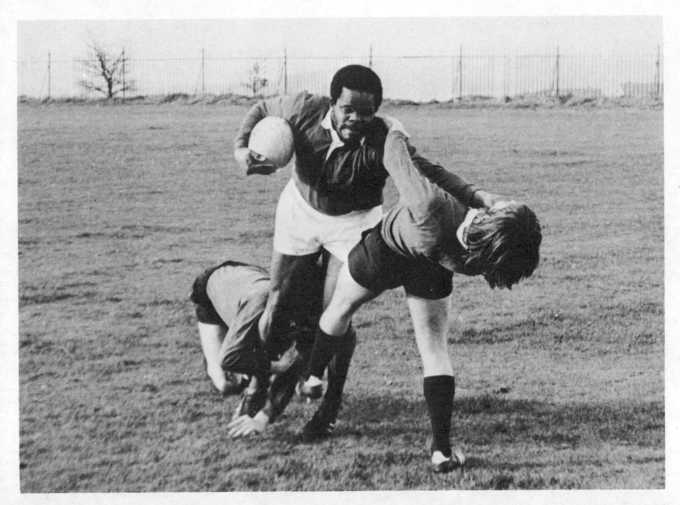

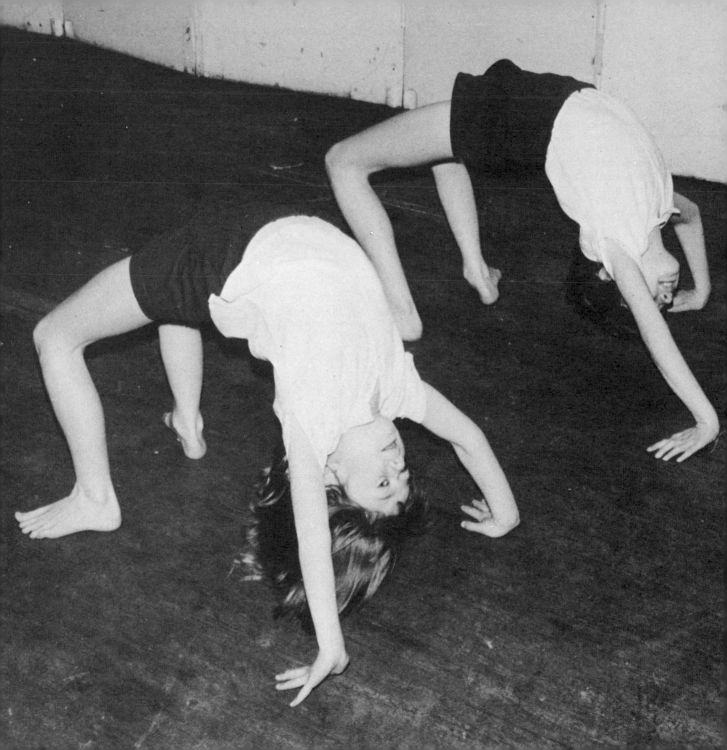

Suppleness of flexibility is to be found in abundance in young children, such as the two illustrated here, but it decreases as people grow older and all sportsmen need to exercise to improve flexibility.

Flexibility

(also referred to as "mobility" and "suppleness")

This quality refers to the suppleness of an individual's body, the ability to flex and extend the muscles and limbs fully. This ability to move the arms or legs or spine through a great range of movement is found in differing degrees among sports participants. It is generally accepted that women are more supple than men. But an examination of sportsmen shows that swimmers and gymnasts tend to possess the most all-round flexibility, whereas footballers and other games players tend to be the most stiff. Weight-lifters usually possess great flexibility, thus exploding the myth of "muscle-bound" properties of strength work.

There seems to be conflict even among experts about whether it is the muscles, joint capsules or ligaments that are stretched by exercises. Evidence is available that flexibility can be improved, therefore it is justifiable to assume that a greater range of movement can be acquired for sportsmen and that this greater range will enable them to apply force over a greater range. That is to say, increased all-round flexibility can improve a person's speed, for it can enable him to apply force on the ground over a greater period of time, and enable his arms to drive through a greater range. It can also be safely assumed that increased flexibility in the legs can enable a person to kick a ball further, because of the increased range through which his leg could move while applying force to the ball. Additionally, it can be said that a greater range of flexibility in the shoulders and arms enables the throwing of an object to a greater

tance. Thus sportsmen should aim to maintain all-round flexibility so that their sporting performances can be improved, for it has also been established that flexibility is lost through ageing and lack of exercise. Generally, the flexibility exercises can be incorporated as part of a sportsman's warm-up, thus a regular routine ensures that no particular area of the body is neglected. Such routines are described in a later chapter.

Skill

". . . behaviour that tends to eliminate the discrepancy between intention and performance."

R. C. Oldfield, *New Biology*, **13**, 1952

When we watch the performance of a pole-vaulter clearing a bar set at 18 feet, we gaze with admiration at his skilful performance. Normally we do this because we know we cannot pole-vault well ourselves. The pole-vaulter has an ability that we do not possess. There are many other situations in which that particular pole-vaulter himself might similarly admire the sporting performances of others, e.g. high-diving, tennis, golf or horse-riding. The very able pole-vaulter would thus be aware that *he* was observing abilities which he did not possess. Thus when we consider **skill**, we must realise that people may in fact be skilful in one sporting situation but useless in another, e.g. a top-class shot-putter can be a non-swimmer.

We should never therefore expect a person to become more skilful at, say, high jumping unless his training includes high jump practice. But a further warning needs to be expressed here, that of the conditions in which the training takes place. If the high jumper practises high-jump technique repeatedly over a bar set at 5 ft 6 in., he will become a very good high jumper over 5 ft 6 in. But should he wish to improve his standard of performance, he would need to raise the bar in training to greater heights.

Frequently we see wasteful practices in training sessions. In football, we see players passing the ball to one another in static formations, whereas the actual game consists of movement around the field, *and opposition* attempting to intercept the ball. For skill improve-ment to take place, the practices should be in as near the actual game or competition situation as possible. Some examples include:

(a) Sprinters should not use starting blocks to run out a few metres in order to improve their start. They should run flat out for about fifty metres trying to beat someone who is sprinting alongside.

(b) Golf players should not simply practice their swings in their back gardens. For improvement, they need to go to hit golf balls, aiming for a particular distance in a particular direction.

(c) Football players should not only play football games as part of their training, because the team consists of a number of different players who need to improve their own ability in a number of different situations. Therefore games situations can be broken

The international athlete here is demonstrating a good starting position for sprinting, but often schoolboys would be better occupied *not* attempting to emulate the styles of seniors, because their strength, speed and skill ability is present in different proportions. Unfortunately, coaches tend to believe that there is only one way of performing a particular skill.

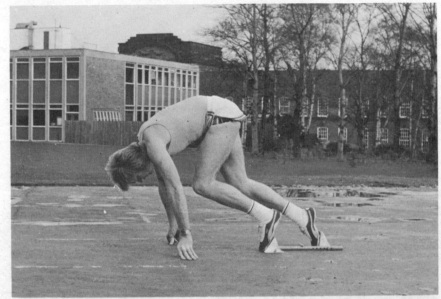

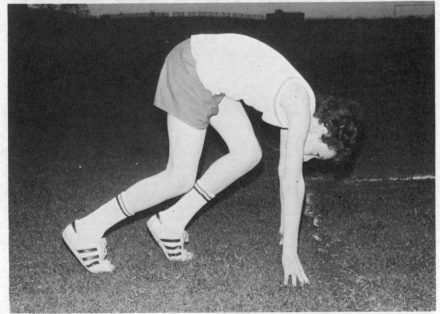

down and practised in twos, threes, fours etc., as well as providing opportunities for the individuals and the whole team to improve.

Performances in sporting activity consist of many skills, and ability at these skills will improve only after lengthy, regular practice. But coaches should avoid the danger (a) of providing useless practices, and (b) neglecting the other components of strength, endurance, etc.

Coaches tend to sit at the edge of the games field thinking that they are doing a lot of good shouting instructions to their players, whereas in fact their players either cannot hear the instructions or are unable to carry them out anyway.

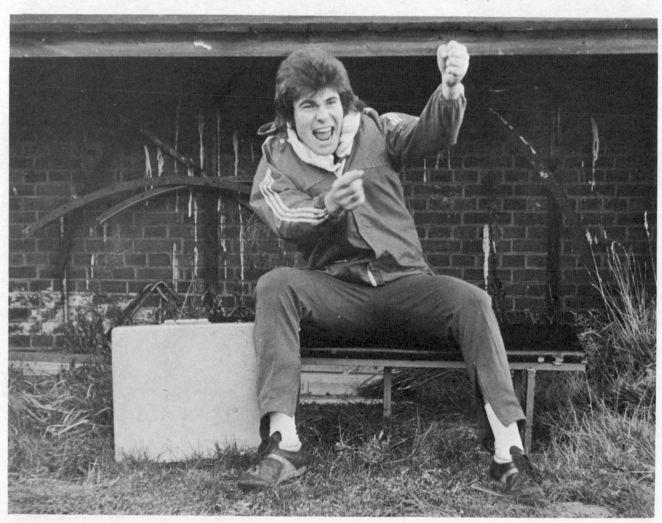

Psychological Factors

"Coaching is 80% kidology."

Anon.

Many of us know of excellent sportsmen who, when they were schoolchildren, were potential world-beaters, but who failed to "make the grade" in the hurly-burly of top-class sport. We also know of many top-class sportsmen who play well in their own team near home, or whose individual performances near home are of the highest calibre, but who fail to reproduce this form at international level.

Usually a sportsman can perform best in familiar surroundings, when the spectators are willing him to succeed, and when he has his own coach nearby. Even world record-holders in sports such as swimming and track and field athletics have reacted differently in front of foreign crowds when the psychological pressure is at its highest, and in fact have been beaten by performances well below their own world-record. On the other hand, some sportsmen seem to need tougher competition to "pull" the best out of them. Usually, coaches tend to discuss such situations under the heading of "motivation", and this simply refers to the reasons, influences or inducements that affect sportsmen's performances.

Some coaches regard the psychological aspect of sport as a relatively unimportant one, or one that can be served simply by shouting at the players in training or during their actual sporting performances. The situation in fact is far more complex. Admittedly, some sportsmen **do** react well to abuse from coaches, but some sportsmen **do not.** As was pointed out earlier in this book, each sportsman and woman is a different person, who physiologically **and** psychologically needs **different treatment.** A later chapter of this book illustrates the different psychological approaches needed by different sportsmen and women, and methods are suggested by which coaches can ascertain which players need which particular approach.

Warm-up

Warming-up

Before any bouts of vigorous sporting activity, it is usual to prepare the muscles by gentle exercise. The reasons for this are justified differently by various coaches and sportsmen, but seem generally to come under three main headings:
(a) to prevent injury,
(b) to improve performance, and
(c) as a psychological preparation.
(a) Those who consider that warming-up is an injury-prevention measure point out that when a muscle or group of muscles around a joint contract (the protagonists), the opposing group of muscles on the other side of the joint (the antagonists) need to lengthen. Often injuries occur in the "antagonists" because they have not lengthened sufficiently to allow the vigorous contracting of the 'protagonist' muscles. An obvious example of this is the injury to "hamstring" muscles at the back of the thigh—the type of injury incurred during vigorous lift of the leg during sprinting. For this reason, some coaches would say that the muscles about to be used should be **gradually** put through the movements until a full-out effort can be made without risk of injury. There are of course researchers who have shown that when observing sportsmen training without warm-up over a period of time, no injuries were incurred. But to assume that this indicates that warm-up is unnecessary would be an error of judgement, because a variety of factors has to be taken into account, not the least being the climate. In very cold weather, it could be folly to indulge in explosive muscular activity without gentle jogging and stretching beforehand.
(b) Those who are of the opinion that warming-up is an aid to improve performance illustrate their belief by comparing the body with a motor-car. They observe that one would not go into a garage early in the morning and expect a cold car to be driven away at 100 m.p.h. Similarly, they would claim the body needs a short time of adjustment before it becomes most efficient. Some researchers have suggested that the body is most efficient when the pulse-rate is between 120 and 180 beats per minute, and that preparatory work is required to bring the body up to 120 beats.
(c) Many coaches and athletes regard the warm-up as psychological preparation for the competition or game ahead. It presents an opportunity for the individual to "gather his wits", concentrate his thoughts on the task ahead, mentally rehearse the routines that he is about to perform, and at world-class level to induce a form of self-hypnosis so that he is oblivious to all that is going on around him that might interfere with or distract him from performing at his best.
Finally, it should be said that whatever the reasons may be, the

most successful sportsmen and sportswomen always warm-up before their training and competitions.

The following exercises are some that have been found to be useful all-round "stretchers", and form a beneficial routine prior to training or competition.

Flexibility Exercises

The kind of warm-up that a person does depends upon his sport. Generally, it will consist of 400 to 1,500 metres jogging followed by some muscle-stretching exercises, then some brief explosive vigorous activity. **Warm-up is also essential before training sessions.** During this period of 15 to 30 minutes, exercises may be used that concentrate on specific weaknesses of the individual, e.g. he may well be stiff in the shoulders, so some arm stretching work will be done; if he is stiff in the legs, some leg-muscle stretching would be included; or it could be a stiffness in the back, so some "spine-stretching" activity would be included.

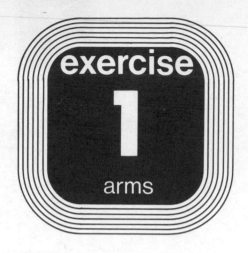

exercise 1
arms

ARM CIRCLING

The starting position is with the arms held straight down in front of the body, the feet close together. Note that the games player prefers to train with bare legs. Normally track suit bottoms should be worn during the warm-up.

Slowly, the arms—kept straight and stiff—are pushed well in front of the body and up into the air as high as possible. At the same time the body rises on to the tiptoes, the arms brush the ears. The position is held for 2–3 seconds.

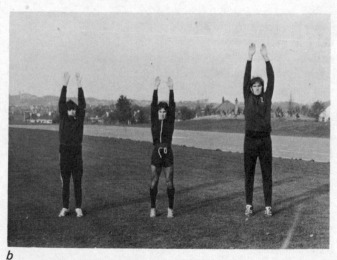

a

b

28

Then the arms are pressed as far behind the back as possible and slowly descend sideways, with the emphasis on keeping the shoulder blades together, until the starting position is again reached. The body weight is lowered onto the heels again.

This exercise is good for men, women and children and can be repeated 6–10 times.

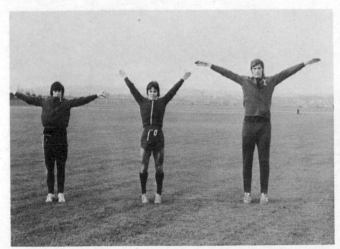

c

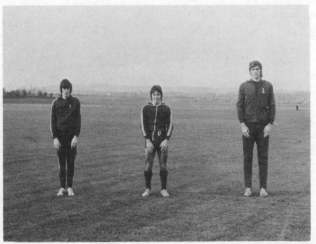

d

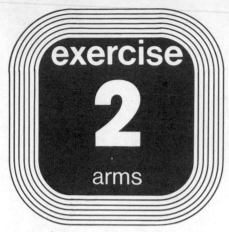

exercise 2
arms

TRUNK BEND, HANDS CLAP

The starting position is with the feet wide apart, the trunk bending forward, hands shoulder-width apart.

a

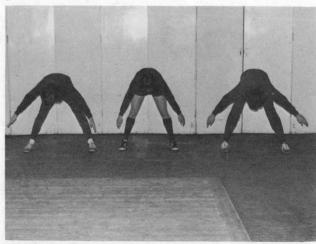

The hands are clapped in front of the body, while the legs and trunk remain in the same position.

b

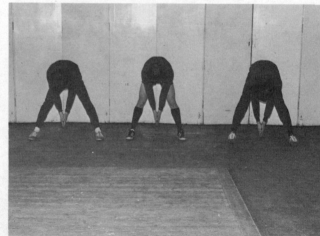

The arms are swept upwards and
backwards.

c

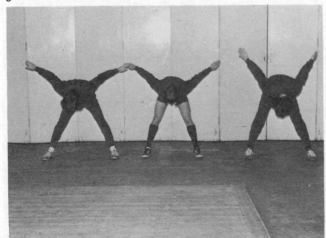

The hands are clapped behind the
body and the arms return to the
starting position.

It is a safe, useful activity for men
and women of all ages and can be
repeated 6–10 times.

d

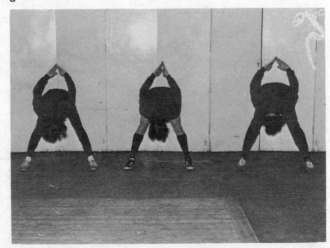

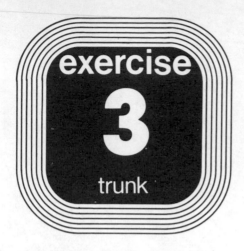

exercise 3 trunk

TRUNK CIRCLING

The starting position is with the feet at shoulder-width or wider apart and hands clasped in front of the body.

a

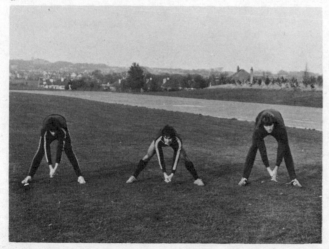

The arms are pressed far away from the body slowly to the side.

b

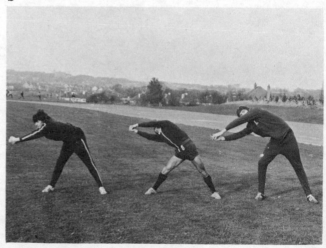

The arms continue in a slow sweep outwards and upwards with the hands being pushed as far away from the body as possible and the trunk leaning as far back as possible without overbalancing.

c

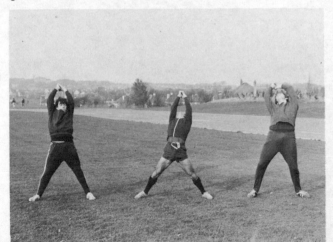

The arms are slowly lowered to the beginning again. Then the exercise is repeated going back in the opposite direction.

It is a good exercise for all, and should be repeated 6–10 times.

d

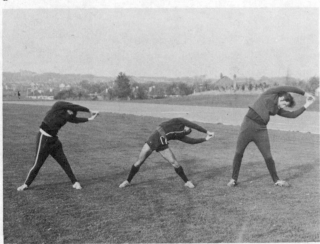

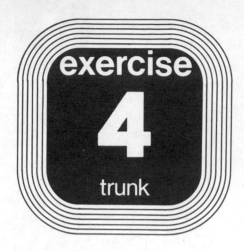

exercise 4 trunk

CRAB

The starting position is lying on the back, flat of the feet on the floor and hands on the floor behind the head.

a

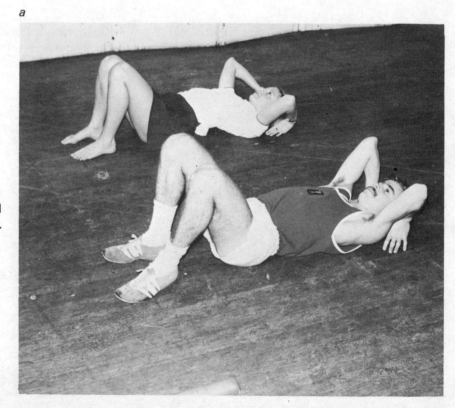

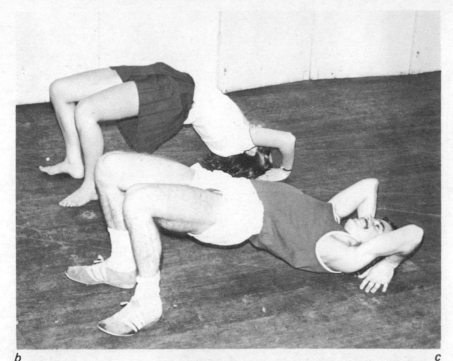

Gently and slowly the body is pushed from the floor until the abdomen is as high in the air as possible, the hands and feet bearing the body weight. Note the stiffness of the man compared with the woman.

b   c

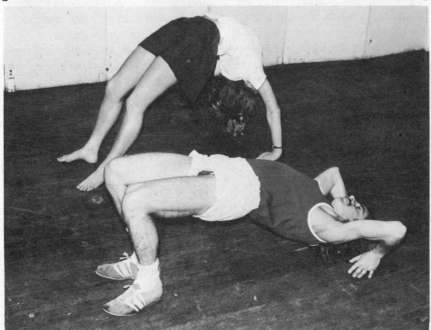

The position is held for 2–3 seconds, then the body is lowered again.

It is a difficult exercise for some people (though children and women are more likely to be sufficiently supple to do it). Those who find it difficult are those who need to do it, i.e. they are too weak or too stiff. It should not be indulged in to the extent of too much strain, but should be attempted more frequently and with the body raised higher at each attempt until eventually 6–10 times in good form is achieved.

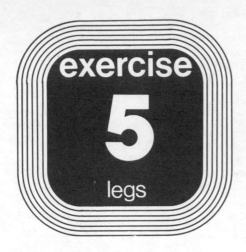

exercise 5
legs

HURDLE POSITION

Sitting on the floor, one leg is moved back until the heel touches the buttock and there is as near to a 90° angle between the thighs as possible. The two games players (on the right) find this difficult.

Slowly and gently, the arms are pushed forward until the hands touch the foot in front and the head touches the knee. Note the basketball player on the left, though supple in the hips, is stiff in the spine.

The exercise can be repeated with the other leg in front.

Those who are stiff in the legs (often the games players) should attempt this, but should not jerk into the exercise. It must be a slow, sustained push forward of the arms and head. Eventually, one should be able to complete the exercise on each leg about 6 times.

a

b

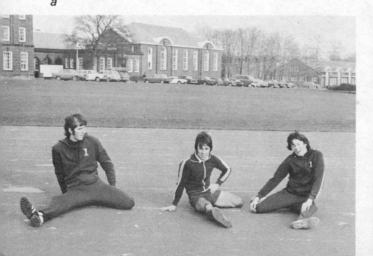

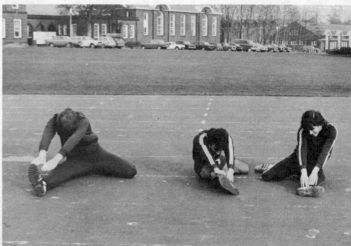

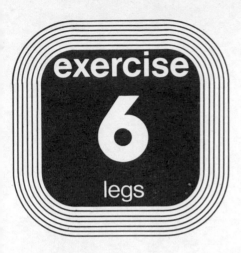

exercise 6 legs

HAMSTRING STRETCH

The starting position is with the outside of the feet touching.

Gently the body is lowered so that the hands either touch the toes, or the hands are placed flat on the ground

The body is then raised up again and the exercise is repeated by alternately having right and left leg in front.

It is a useful exercise for all, but it must not be carried out in a jerky fashion.

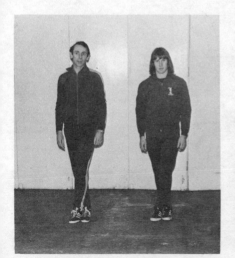

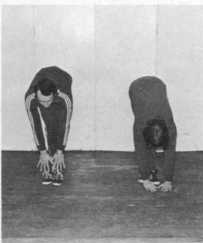

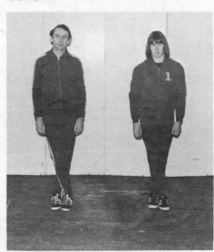

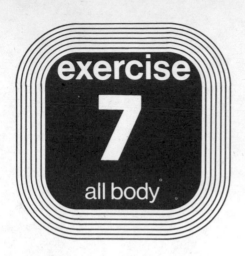

exercise 7
all body

KNEE TO CHEST

The exercises so far have been of a slow, stretching, nature. Before practising the actual skill of the individual's sport, a more explosive activity is required using the whole of the body.

With feet close together, the sportsman jumps high up into the air so that **his knees touch his chest.**

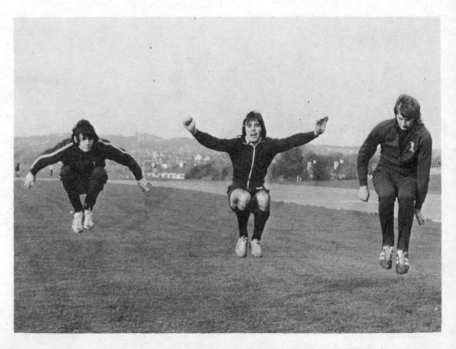

The exercise can be repeated 6–10 times.

The next stage is the actual training session, or the game. The volume of work carried out in the warm-up will depend upon the weather (in hot weather, less warm-up is necessary), the sport, and the nature of the competition. In some instances, sportsmen will take a rest *after* the warm-up, perhaps for the purpose of bringing the pulse rate down a little; or for the opportunity to collect the mental processes together before the competition, or simply for administrative reasons such as collecting equipment together.

Then the athlete is ready for his running, endurance, or strength activity.

Planning Running Schedules

Distance Running

Running very long distances in training is essential—for long distance runners! But these kind of training sessions need to be used only sparingly for most other sportsmen. Those coaches who advocate regular long-distance road runs or cross-country runs should, in the author's opinion, do two things. First, they should **accompany** their sportsmen on these regular runs. Secondly, if they are still convinced of their value, they should recall the speed at which they ran the distance and ascertain how many times, during the game in which they have an interest, the players run at that speed.

Long-distance jogs during the pre-season or early season training are a most effective way of bringing players gently back from a state of unfitness to one where they are ready for the more severe strains of hard training. But long-distance

runs take a lot of precious time; often they are unpopular; sportsmen can cheat by not putting in the effort when not in sight, and it is difficult to ensure that the participants are getting the correct benefit from them. They **do** ensure an improvement in circulatory-respiratory endurance if carried out correctly. They **can** be a relief from the boredom occasionally brought on by training at the same games-field, track etc. They can also be introduced as a challenging team or individual competition. But these advantages must be weighed against the advantages derived from other types of running training.

Analysing the Running Requirements of a Game

In major team games, e.g. football, rugby, hockey, cricket, basketball etc., coaches often find it difficult to ascertain how to devise fitness schedules that will enable the players to receive the appropriate amount of running or circulo-respiratory endurance work. Frequently, coaches depend on their own judgment in giving an arbitrary amount of sprinting, jogging and cross-country work. But most will agree that they would prefer a more accurate guide.

The author and some of his students have attempted to analyse the running requirements of **different players in the same game** (not just the "average" type of running that the players would perform). The results of a soccer study are printed below Table 1. Coaches could copy the method of analysis in their

Table 1

Soccer Full-back's Work Rate

(in metres)

	Sprinting	Striding	Jogging	Walking	Totals
Leeds United (English Top-class Performers)	2587	2751	3541	2593	11,472
Luton Town (English Second Division)	1514	1971	2817	3984	10,286
Hitchin (English Top-class Amateurs)	1183	1817	2576	4103	9,679
Carnegie (English College Students)	531	1073	1871	3134	6,609

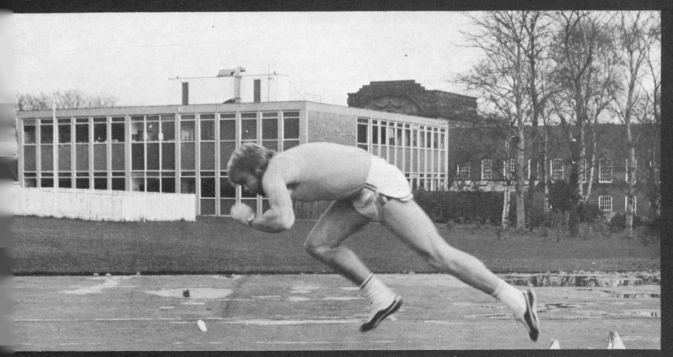

Running fast is an ability with which some are blessed and which some work hard to acquire. But running fast is relative to each particular sport and sportsmen should analyse the type of running required by *them* and not simply emulate the work done by those in other sports, e.g. as illustrated here by an international athlete. He is simply demonstrating the type of running needed not by international athletes, but specifically only by those who need to use starting blocks.

Table 2
Soccer Half-back's Work Rate
(in metres)

	Sprinting	Striding	Jogging	Walking	Totals
Leeds United (English Top-class Performers)	1891	2288	4607	5041	13,827
Luton Town (English Second Divisiion)	1001	1091	4178	4914	11,184
Hitchin (English Top-class Amateurs)	912	942	3404	3826	9084
Carnegie (English College Students)	873	1348	2971	3562	8754

own games. The method divided the moving about of players into WALKING (forwards, backwards and sideways), JOGGING (including skipping in different directions, that is moving about at faster than "walking" pace), STRIDING (meaning over half-speed, covering more ground at each pace than "jogging") and SPRINTING (obviously meaning running or moving at flat-out speed). A player's game was analysed in this manner, by counting the number of paces he took at the speeds described. Afterwards, during a training session the player's stride-length at walking, jogging, striding and sprinting were measured. Thus the distance he covered throughout a game could be calculated.

It will be noted that players in the *same position* but for different teams of different levels of ability cover different distances during a game. Thus the printing of fitness programmes for, say, "footballers"

would be a wasteful occupation. It also indicates that players of different *positions* might also cover different distances, therefore the analysis of players of a different position from that illustrated in Table 1 are reproduced in Table 2 for comparison.

The implication is that running programmes should be devised to include different speeds i.e. not only sprinting, not only long-distance slow runs, but a mixture of these and other types of running. The running activities, as in games, should include changes of direction, sideways and backward running, and occasionally running with the ball. But not **all** work should be done with the ball at the players' feet or in their hands, or with racquets, bats etc. For the introduction of equip-

ment tends to slow the player down, thus reducing the rate of improvement of his speed or endurance factor.

Gaining the extra yard of speed

Games players, athletes and coaches are always looking for methods to make them that "extra yard faster". If they were to consider the problem carefully, the mystery would begin to be cleared up, for so many rely on gimmicks as opposed to sensible solutions to their predicament.

If "speed off the mark" is a requirement, the coach is asking for his player to be more readily able to project his body weight in a particular direction at a given moment. That is, he is admitting that his player is not strong enough to cope more adequately with his present body weight. In this case, the player should reduce his weight, or improve his strength. But if the coaches, or athletes, are anxious for this faster movement to continue not only one or two paces but say up

to 50 metres, or 30 metres, then speed, endurance **and** skill come into the picture.

Running fast is a **skill** that needs to be practised just as other skills are. A person's ability to throw snowballs at a target will improve as the winter progresses when the person has had more practice at throwing snowballs. The skill will fall off during the summer when the opportunity to throw snowballs is not present. Similarly, running fast must be practised. It will not improve through practising at $\frac{3}{4}$ speed with a ball at the feet, or a ball in the hand. In many games the players' running is predominantly **without** the ball for most of the game anyway. Therefore sportsmen and women who wish to improve speed and "getting quick off the mark" should practise those activities. The following are the kind of activities that could be used during training sessions, but need not constitute the whole of the session.

Short Sprints

(a) Standing with a foot on a line, preferably with another person alongside, a useful practice is to race 30 metres with the emphasis on vigorous *arm* drive and the knees coming up vigorously and high. Walk back to the starting point and repeat another five times. Take two or three minutes rest and repeat the six sprints, followed by a further short rest, then a further six sprints, another rest, then six sprints. This is usually referred to as 4 sets of 6 repetitions with a 2 or 3 minute rest between (or 4 × 6, 30 metres). The rest between sets allows sufficient recovery to enable the practice to be one of **sprinting** and not an **endurance** exercise.

(b) A method of avoiding the boredom of repeating the same activity for about 24 times as in (a) above is to vary the distance run, i.e. those training could be required to sprint 20 metres, then after walking back to the start they could sprint 30 metres, then 40 metres, 50 metres, then finally 60 metres. At this point a 2 to 3 minutes rest period would be appropriate. In the next group set, the distances could be reversed i.e. first the 60 metres, then 50 metres, 40 metres, 30 metres and 20 metres finally. After a further short rest, 20, 30, 40, 50 and 60 metres; rest; then 60, 50, 40 30, 20 metres sprints. This method is known as "up and down the clock" work. It enables athletes to have a reducing distance to run when they are becoming tired, thus psychologically ensuring that the effort is not reduced.

(c) A team practice that includes speed work is a "continuous relay". In this, those who are assembled are divided into teams of seven, eight, nine or ten members (not necessarily equal teams). They are then spread at equal distances around a track, football field or similar perimeter of approximately 400 metres. On a signal from the coach/trainer, the first in each team runs fast to hand a piece of wood (or relay baton) to their second in the team, he then runs to the third etc. **But,** in handing over the baton, each runner remains on the track because the last runner will hand the baton to the first man etc. so that all teams will cover a *number* of laps.

The coach might inform the teams at the beginning that the race will be of, say, 6 laps duration (i.e. each member will be sprinting 6 × 40 or 50 metres), or he might make it a 10-minute race—the team in front after 10 minutes being the winners. The competitive element in such races makes the participants put in full effort.

(d) One of the common reasons why sportsmen and women are slower than they need to be is the fact that they are not aware of the importance of the use of the upper body as well as the legs to obtain speed. A useful practice to include in training sessions is that of setting a distance of about 20 metres (in football, the 18 yards line will do, in rugby the 25 yards line, in athletics the 20 metres relay box). Those training should be required to stand with one foot on a line then sprint the short distance about six times *attempting to cover the distance in the fewest strides possible*—with emphasis on arms. This practice three or four times during a session would eventually result in the arms and shoulders being used more efficiently during the normal game situation.

Running for Endurance

Most of the activities listed as "speed" practices can become endurance work if the rest between is cut, so that for instance a person is required to *jog* back after each sprint instead of *walking* back. But additional methods may be used to ensure the improvement of circulo-respiratory endurance:

(a) An excellent activity that improves endurance is hill or sand-dune running. Ideally, a steep hill of at least 100 metres should be sought for this purpose. Those training would be required to sprint up the hill with a gap of about five metres between individuals. On reaching the top, they should walk down, then sprint up again—repeating the run about six times and attempting to ensure that they are not being overtaken by those behind them.

This could be followed by their skill work, or it could be half of a fitness session used after, say, their light sprint session.

(b) Rather than using a 5000 metres run at a moderate speed, most games players would benefit from an overall slightly shorter distance broken down into faster runs, i.e. 3 sets of 5 repetitions of 100 metres (total 1500) run in the following fashion:
Those training should be lined up in groups of three or four and should sprint 100 metres, *jog back;* sprint 100 metres, etc., 5 times. After about 3 minutes rest, a further 5 sprints; 3 minutes rest; then a final 5 sprints. The distances could be modified according to the needs of the sportsmen. But sprinting with a jog back recovery is far more beneficial than long runs.

(c) As in speed work, "up and down the clock" runs are valuable in the building up of endurance, e.g: sprint 30 metres, jog back; sprint 40 metres, jog back; sprint 50 metres, jog back; sprint 60 metres, jog back; sprint 70 metres, jog back. This could be repeated three or four times, each group being different from the previous, i.e. if the first were an "up the clock" series, the next would be down, etc.

(d) Team runs over distances of 2 to 3 miles are often more beneficial than individual races of twice the distance because extra effort may be put into a race to uphold the honour of the team. For instance, the group training could be divided into small teams of three or four sportsmen. The race distance would be chosen and described. The men would be required to cover this distance over different types of terrain, and on returning the positions that they came in the race would be totalled. The team obtaining the *LOWEST* total would win e.g.:

TEAM A	TEAM B	TEAM C
1st man back	4th man back	2nd man back
7th man back	5th man back	3rd man back
9th man back	6th man back	8th man back
TOTALS 17	15	13

Therefore Team C wins, Team B is second, Team A is last.

(e) Another useful endurance training session may be carried out by those groups whose trainer goes with them! The course should be planned to cover all types of countryside, and the run organised on the "fartlek" principle, i.e. Scandinavian "speed-play". The trainer would jog with his sportsmen for about 800 metres, then he might require them to sprint 100 metres, then walk 100 metres, jog 100 metres, skip 100 metres, run backwards 50 metres, run sideways 50 metres, walk 100 metres, sprint 100 metres, etc., over a distance of 5000 or 10,000 metres (3–6 miles). The run could also be interspersed with periods during which press-ups, squat jumps, or other exercises could be included if the terrain happened to be flat. In the event of a hilly course being selected, there might appear to be sufficient variety of exercise in climbing over fences and running up steep hills for other exercises not to be included.

Whatever types of running that coaches/trainers decide is appropriate for the sportsmen in their care, the important features that need to be emphasised are that the training runs must not be boring; that variety of types of running must be included; and most important of all they must be designed to have a particular effect. That is to say, coaches must know *and should let the sportsmen know* for what purpose the running is included. Purposeless long runs will not necessarily improve endurance. Enjoyable hard running sessions that differ in nature each day and that have an occasional element of competition are more likely to improve endurance.

Planning Muscular Endurance Sessions

Circuit Training

In 1957, a book was published which gave details of a method of training recently devised by G. T. Adamson and R. E. Morgan, two lecturers in physical education at the University of Leeds. The book, *Circuit Training*, stated that the method essentially aims at "the development of all-round fitness rather than the fitness required for any particular game or activity".

Since that time, "circuit training" has been modified to suit the needs of most sports, and it is an essential feature of muscular endurance training. The advantages in using circuit training are numerous and include:

(a) it contains a great variety of different exercises to satisfy all sports participants,
(b) it does not take a great deal of time,
(c) each participant (and the coach) can see his own progress as the weeks progress,
(d) participants can work at their own rate without being supervised in all that they do,
(e) it can be carried out in a confined space,
(f) If a gymnasium is used, hundreds can train in the space of one evening,
(g) it is accurately planned for each individual's needs, and
(h) it can be carried out indoors during those periods of the year when bad weather prevents outside training.

In the author's experience, it is generally accepted as an enjoyable form of training, an effective means of acquiring muscular endurance, easily organised even with large numbers, **and a very useful method of indicating whether a sportsman has completely recovered after injury.**

The actual exercises used can be modified to suit the needs of specialist groups, as can the number of exercises and the lengths of time of the tests. This present chapter gives details, based on circuit sessions organised by the author for college and university students who were training for a number a different sports.

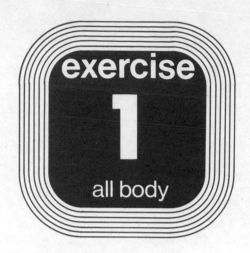

Selection of Exercises

For mature students and sportsmen, the author has observed that ten exercises appears to be adequate, though for women and schoolchildren this number can be reduced to eight (or alternatively their target time can be reduced; this is dealt with later).

The ten exercises selected are normally organised so that no similar muscle groups are concentrated upon in consecutive exercises. As far as possible, exercises are selected for arms, follow by abdominals, then legs, with occasional exercises combining all three main areas of the body. The actual exercise will depend upon the facilities and equipment available, and the layout of the room in which the circuit training is to take place. The general principle of mixing the exercises should be adopted where possible.

BENCH LIFTS

This exercise, demonstrated by a top-class triple jumper, commences with a gymnasium bench hooked on the wallbars at a height of about 6 to 7 feet. The individual grasps the free end of the bench near to his chest in a full squat position.

He then begins to stand up, raising the bench.

Then the bench is raised as high over the head as possible, with the body also being raised onto the tiptoes.

Finally, he squats down to the floor again.

This, and other exercises, should be carried out in a fast rhythmic (not jerky) fashion.

International women athletes have coped with this exercise adequately, though some weaker women prefer not to raise the bench high above their heads, nor to squat so low.

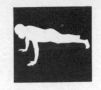

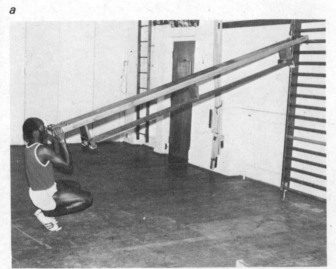

a

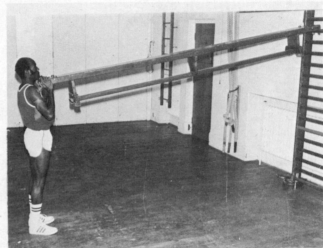

b

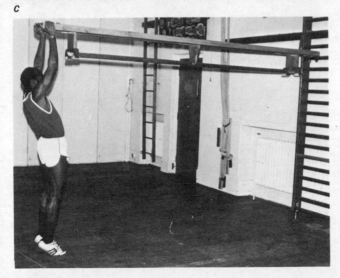

c

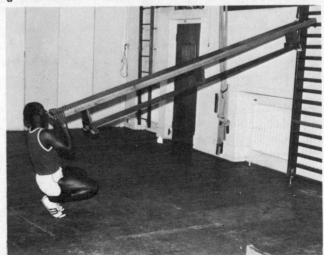

d

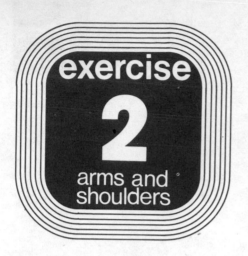

exercise

2

arms and
shoulders

CHINS

This activity exercises mainly the arm and shoulder muscles and is performed on a beam or similar bar. This beam or bar must be set at a height which ensures that the person's feet cannot touch the floor when he is holding it.

The starting position is with the person grasping the bar with arms shoulder-width apart and palms in the direction that he is facing (here, an international gymnast demonstrates). The body must be permitted to hang freely and motionless before the activity commences.

The person then pulls up the body by the use of effort in arms and shoulders, without kicking, swinging or jerking the lower body. When he touches the beam or bar with his chin, he may then lower his body again.

The exercise is complete when the body is lowered in a fully extended position, with the arms perfectly straight again and the body still.

For women, this exercise may be modified by placing the bar at a height that the individual can just reach when the feet are on the floor. The exercise is then one of jumping **and pulling with the arms,** so that the chin touches the bar.

a
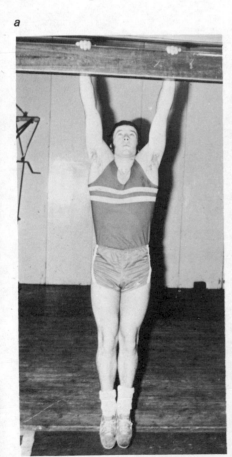

b
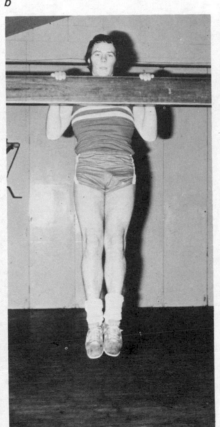

c
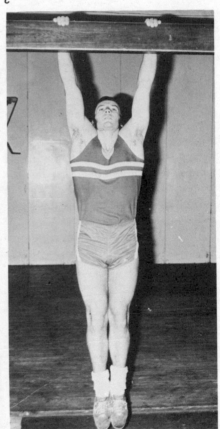

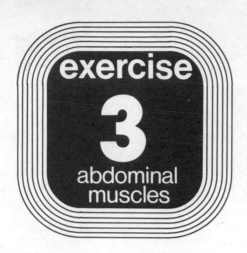

exercise 3 abdominal muscles

TRUNK TWISTS

In this activity, one lies down, hands clasped behind the head, with feet under a bench, bottom wall bar, or similar anchorage point (a friend can press down on the ankles). The knees are both slightly bent. Here, a top-class squash player and a woman athlete demonstrate.

a

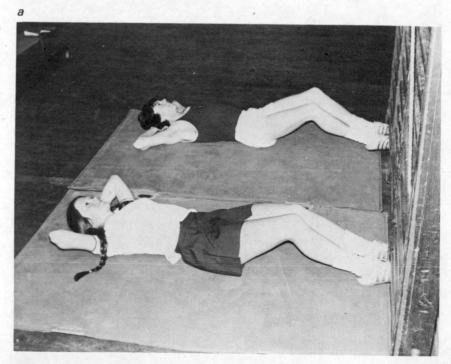

The action is one of raising the body so that the **left** elbow touches the **right** knee.

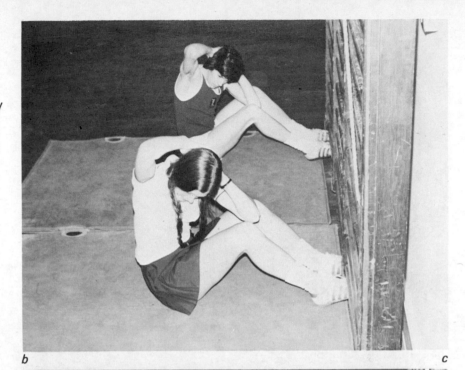

b   c

The body is then lowered to the lying down position.

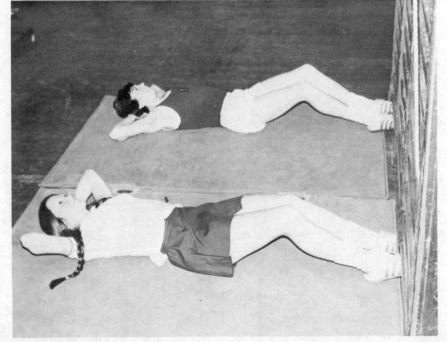

On the next raising of the body, the **right** elbow touches the **left** knee, and so on alternately.
No modifications are necessary for women.

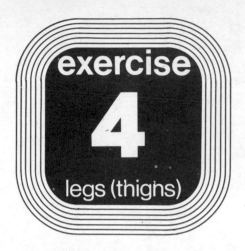

exercise 4
legs (thighs)

SQUAT JUMPS

The starting position for this exercise is with the individual (a rugby player in this photograph) squatting down with one foot in front of the other, head upright, finger-tips of both hands just touching the floor.

Then there is an explosive leap into the air, while the feet change around in mid-air.

The landing position is one where the other foot is now in front, fingers touch the floor, and head upright.

Women can usually cope with this exercise with no difficulty.

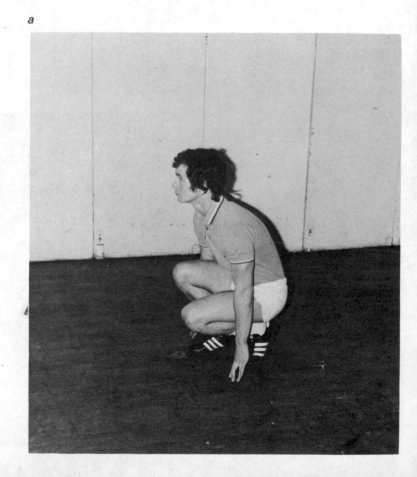

a

54

b

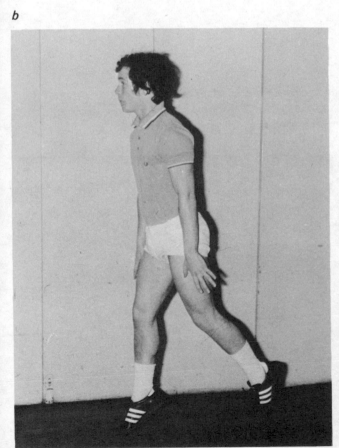

c

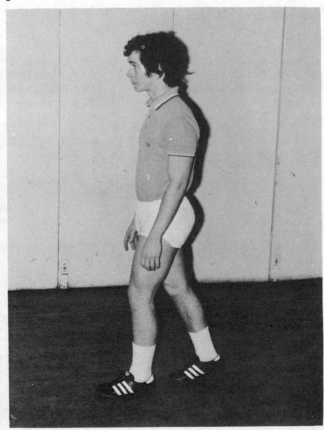

55

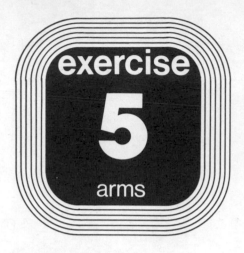

exercise
5
arms

PRESS-UPS

Though mainly an arm exercise, the abdominal, back and leg muscles are also working to keep the body rigid.

The starting position is one where the person (here a top-class baseball player) lies face towards

the floor, palms flat down near the chest with the fingers pointing towards the head.

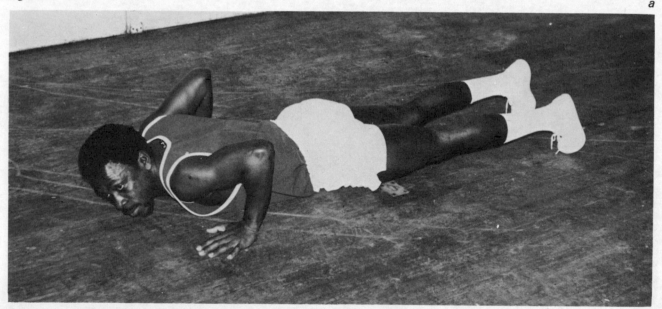

a

The effort comes from the arms, the body being pushed up until the arms are locked at the elbow. The body must not be allowed to sag, neither must the bottom stick up into the air. A straight line from head to toes is the aim.

b

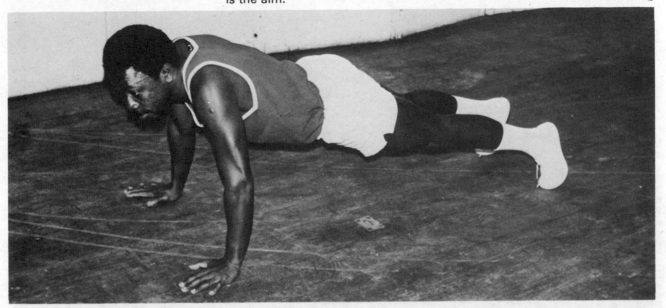

Finally, the body is lowered again

c

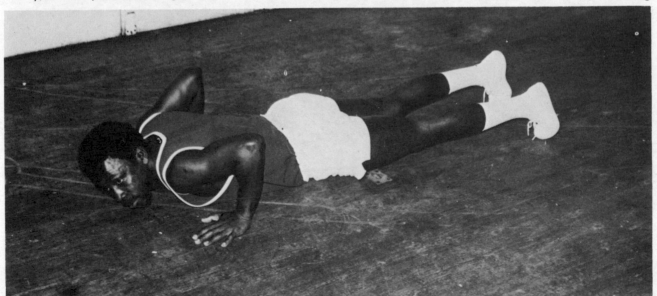

The exercise can be modified for women by permitting them to push up into a kneeling position, then lowering again.

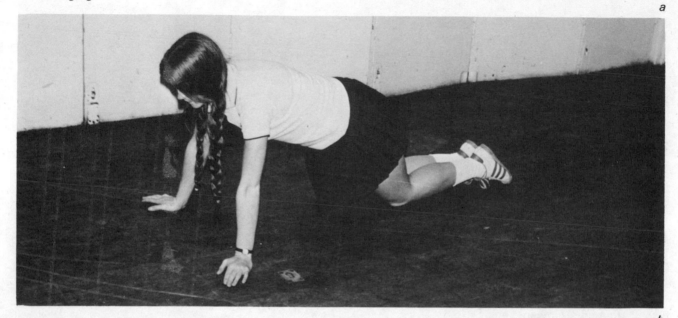

a

b

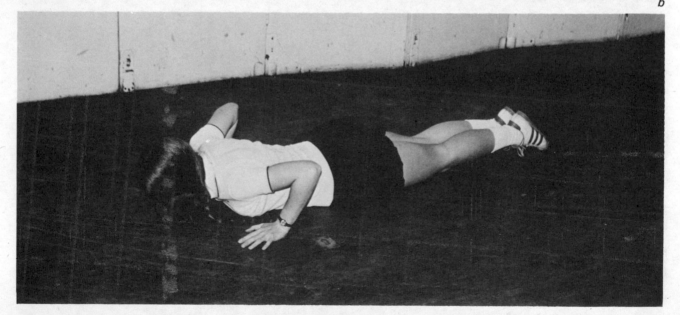

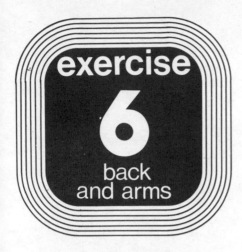

exercise 6
back and arms

CHEAT CURLS

The exercise can be performed with a weight training bar (plus approx. 10 lbs. on each side), or a length of heavy pipe filled with sand, or other heavy object. The bar is grasped with fingers pointing away from the body, and arms are fully extended downwards. The body is erect, feet shoulder-width apart. The demonstrator is an expert tchoukball player.

a

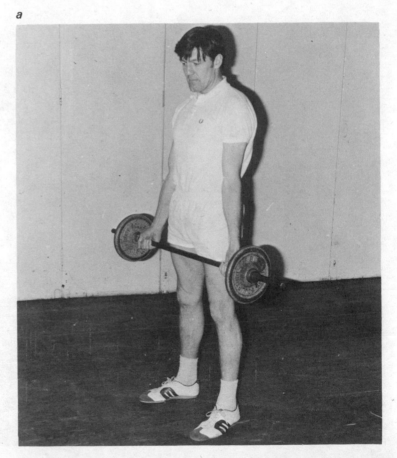

The hips are thrust forward, the body leans back and the weight is pulled towards the chest.

The bar is held momentarily at the chest until the body is upright again.

The bar is then lowered to the legs until the arms are fully extended.

The exercise has been successfully used with women athletes, except that obviously they use lighter weights than men. In some cases for women, the exercise could be carried out with the weight-training bar containing no additional weights.

b

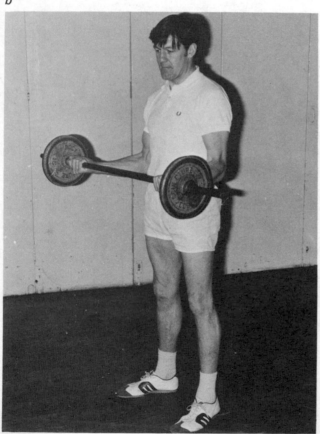

c

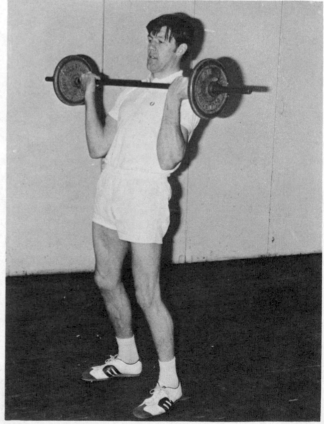

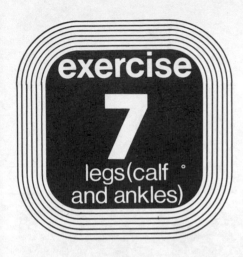

exercise 7
legs(calf and ankles)

ASTRIDE JUMPS

The exercise is begun by standing on the floor astride a 10 in. high bench or solid box. For an active sportsman, this exercise is a relatively easy one unless extra weight is added to his body, e.g. a beam saddle, a pair of dumbells, a medicine ball, etc. Here, a woman inernational swimmer and the author, an international athlete, are shown.

He then jumps down to the starting position again.
The exercise is best performed on the toes and balls of the feet.
Women may use the same exercise without the use of added weights.

Pushing off with the toes of both feet, the sportsman leaps on to the bench.

a

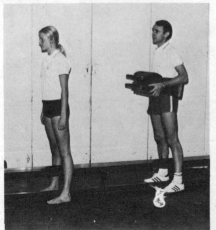

b

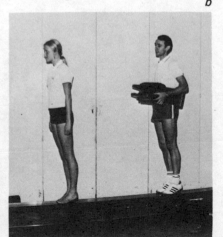

c

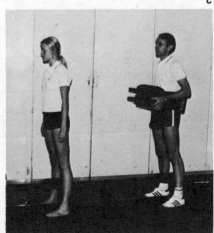

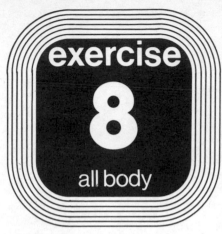

exercise 8
all body

BURPEES

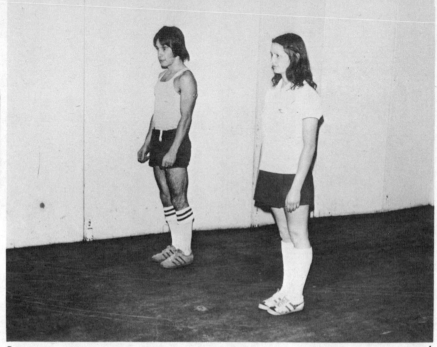

a   b

This is a fast vigorous activity
needing only floor space. The starting position is standing upright, feet
together, hands in front of thighs. A
woman international gymnast and a
male hockey player demonstrate.

Next, a full crouch position is
adopted with the palms flat on the
floor.

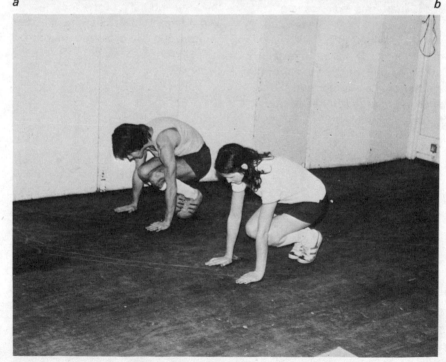

The legs are then shot far back to a full stretched position, hands supporting the body.

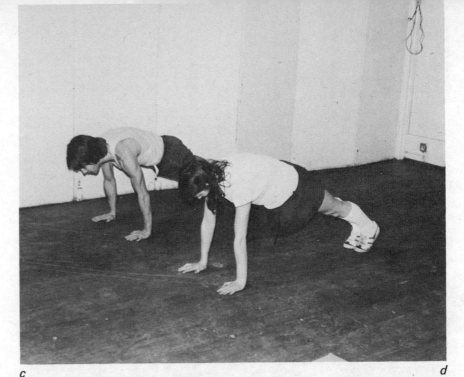

c   d

Then the legs are brought forward to the crouch position once more.

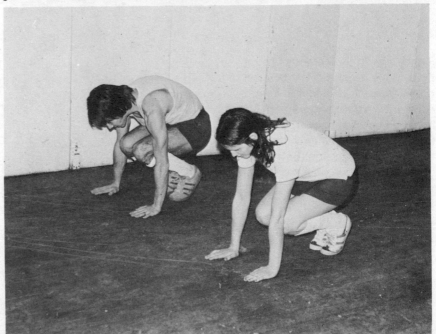

Finally, the athlete stands up-right—this is one complete cycle of the exercise. It is useful to keep a constant rhythm, and trainers can help by shouting ''down, back, forward, up'' in the early stages, so that those performing the exercises do not stay in one position too long.

The activity is perfectly suitable for women.

e

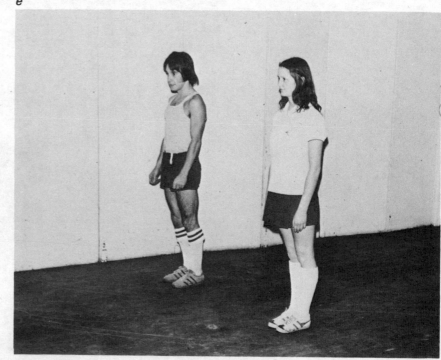

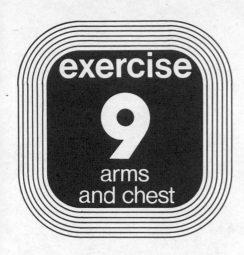

exercise 9
arms and chest

BENT ARM
PULL-OVERS

A comfortable, lying-on-bench position is adopted, here by an Olympic
canoeist, with feet flat on the floor,
and head just resting on the edge of
the bench. A bar with approximately
10 lbs on both ends is on the floor
(or mat) behind the head. This bar is
gripped underneath.

a

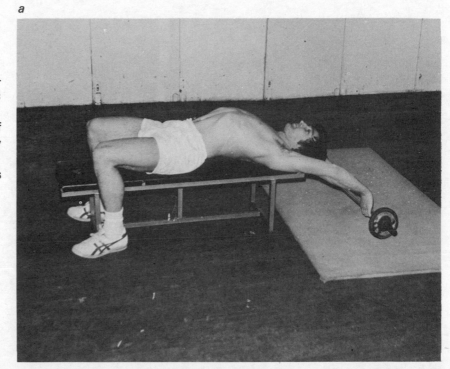

A vigorous pull of the arms raises the bar from the floor. Arms may be bent at this point.

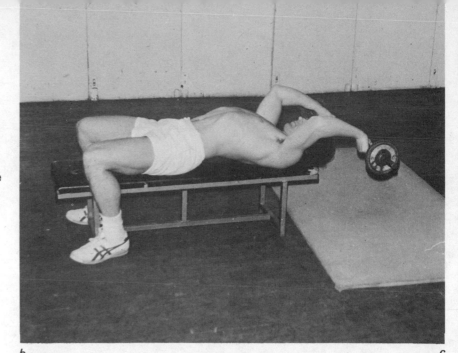

b

c

The bar is then pushed high into the air, arms straight, the weight immediately above the chest.

Finally the bar is slowly lowered behind the head to the floor again with arms bending.

This activity is suitable for women, but with a bar only.
Some sportsmen find difficulty with the exercise owing to stiffness in the shoulder joint. They should commence the exercise with the bar high above the chest and lower behind the head as far as is comfortable. The exercise will in time assist them in overcoming the stiffness.

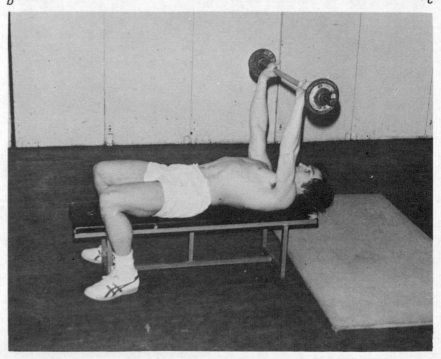

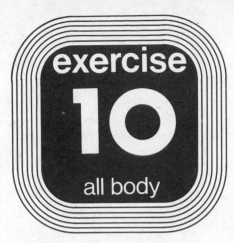

exercise 10
all body

SHUTTLE RUN

One factor important to most sports participants is the ability to "get off the mark" fast and powerfully. Short runs, dodging activities, shuttle runs and other activities including change of direction are therefore of invaluable help. The shuttle run requires fast short runs with the athlete touching the floor with one hand both at the start and at each turning point as illustrated:

It will be observed that in a 60 ft long gymnasium, a run such as illustrated would consist of 100 yards fast running with seven changes of direction. This is of great value to men and women of all sports.

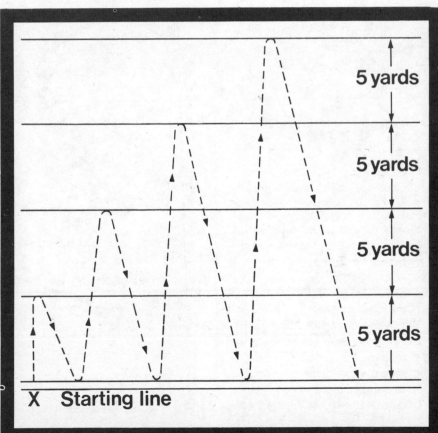

5 yards

5 yards

5 yards

5 yards

X   Starting line

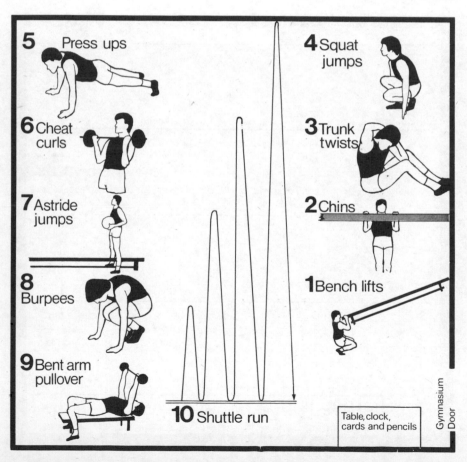

5 Press ups

6 Cheat curls

7 Astride jumps

8 Burpees

9 Bent arm pullover

10 Shuttle run

4 Squat jumps

3 Trunk twists

2 Chins

1 Bench lifts

Table, clock, cards and pencils

Gymnasium Door

Layout of Circuit

The exercises should be well spaced out so that no individual can be injured or impeded by someone working alongside. A circular layout is recommended in a clockwise or anti-clockwise direction, depending upon where the door of the gymnasium or building is situated. (A number of participants generally congregate around the door, either collecting their cards, or entering the time on their cards on completion of the circuit.) A successful layout that has had well over fifty people working at one time is illustrated:

Testing

Each man should be tested to discover his **maximum number of efforts in 60 seconds**, e.g. in "press-ups", he may complete **18** press-ups before becoming fatigued at the 30 seconds point; after a brief rest while lying on the floor, he may be able to complete another **4 press-ups** before the 60 seconds are over. In this case his "score" is **22 press-ups** during the period of 60 seconds. (In the case of women and teenage schoolchildren, it would be advisable to reduce the test time to 30 seconds and/or cut the number of exercises from 10 to a number appropriate to their age and ability.) The testing should be done with the coach or supervisor blowing a whistle at the commencement of the 60-second period; the athletes' scores could be counted by the athlete himself or a fellow-athlete. On completion of each 60-second test, a **2 minute rest** is essential, before the next test.

Preferably, the testing should be done for Exercise No. 1 followed by 2 minutes rest, then Exercise No. 2, etc. In the event of having large numbers, however, the individuals could be spread around the gym so that six or eight individuals would be at each activity, in pairs. One would be working while the other noted his score, then they would change over before passing along to the next exercise. The procedure would be for the timekeeper simply to blow a whistle every 60 seconds. Athlete "A" would work to maximum when the first whistle blew and stop when the second whistle blew, while athlete "B" kept score. On the second whistle athlete "B" would work to maximum until the third whistle, while "A" kept score. After the third whistle, both athletes would enter their scores and move to the next activity. Then when the next (fourth) whistle blows, athlete "A" works to maximum again, etc. Should the testing be done with everyone spread around the gym, the individuals should put their scores on the "circuit cards" under the appropriate column. If Athlete X started his tests on Exercise No. 4, he should be told to start at No. 4 on each occasion he trains in future weeks.

In the circuit described in earlier pages, all exercises **except No. 10** should be tested, i.e. 9 exercises at one minute each, plus 2 minutes rest between each, equals just under a half-hour to organise. Hundreds can therefore be tested in the space of a few hours. Where an organisation has only twenty or thirty players to test, these can easily be catered for in half an hour, after which, if the coach so wishes, other skill practices could form part of the training session.

Circuit Training

On completion of the testing, the situation has arrived where coach, teacher, trainer or athlete has a card with the test 'scores', or maximum performances on 9 activities. The testing is **an occasional, not weekly, procedure**. The next time the person tested arrives at the gym (in most cases circuit training is more appropriately a weekly venture) he should be able to collect his card from a box where all cards are in alphabetical order. On the top of this card appear his name, age, height, weight and main sport (with position played or best performance). His test date and scores will be noted, and in the second row of figures, he will notice (often with some relief) that those figures have been halved. He will be told to make a note of the time and go around the activities performing these half-scores as fast as he can. In the Exercise No. 10 column a figure 1 will appear to indicate that he does the shuttle run once only during one "circuit" of the gymnasium. However, it will be impressed upon him that every circuit training evening, he must do 3 circuits with little or no rest between the 3 x 10 activities. That is to say he times himself doing the half-maximum scores in Exercise 1–10, on completion of this he repeats his half-scores on Exercises 1–10 again, and yet

again a *third* time. On the reverse of his circuit card, he places the time it took him to complete the 3 circuits of the gymnasium, and he leaves the card for the coach's perusal afterwards.

He is **not** permitted to do the half-score of Exercise No. 1 three times, followed by the half-score of Exercise No. 2 three times (thus going around the gymnasium only once). In fact, if he attempted to do that he would be unsuccessful, because his maximum on the test was only 2 x half score!

As a guide the individual can be told that he is expected to complete the **3 "circuits" in under 30 minutes.** Most will be delighted to discover that they do this during the first week, and it provides an incentive for them to return the next week! Once the individual beats a time of **20 minutes,** he must be retested on his next visit. It has been found that between 20 and 30 minutes circuit training is of value to sportsmen;

anything less does not have a great deal of effect on all-round muscular endurance.

Necessary Modifications

The author is aware that facilities such as described are not always available for circuit training. But the examples have been provided as something at which to aim, and most of the exercises can be modified using simple equipment. Exercises Nos. 3, 4, 5, 8 and 10 need no equipment, whereas Exercises Nos. 2, 6, and 7 could also easily be carried out in the open air using goal posts, wooden boxes, tree branches etc. If objections are made to carrying out circuit training outdoors because of inclement weather, the author has organised such training in a football club bar, a refreshment room, club changing rooms, an old horse stable, and in a very large bedroom.

Many coaches will fail to include circuit training in their sessions because it requires initially slick organisation and they cannot be bothered, whereas sportsmen often omit it because it is hard, and it does not hurt so much to spend time on skills sessions instead.

If there are valid reasons for not carrying out circuit training in the form described here, then combined sessions are a useful alternative. These could be used for middle distance runners who sometimes prefer to do half the amount of the 30-minute circuit **after** a road run. Some games teams meet so infrequently that they would claim they cannot devote an evening to circuit training. They too might wish to do a shortened period of circuit training **after** some skills or running activity.

It is contended, however, that in the case of those keen sportsmen who wish to progress, they will find time (in lunch-hours?) to carry out their own circuit training (perhaps around their office desk) regardless of what their team-mates or coaches are doing.

Some clubs organise a system of "beginners", "regulars" and "super" circuits. Others organise a colour system. That is on "chins", the "beginners" or "green" circuit individuals are required to perform 6 of these exercises, whereas the "super" or "red" people perform 12, the intermediate group doing, say, 9. But these are purely arbitrary figures and **can never** be as valuable as the scores derived from the testing of each individual. In some cases, people will be overworked on arms, others on legs, etc. whereas frequently there will be people underworked.

Circuits specifically designed for the needs of football players, or tennis players or other sports participants might include more exercises for muscle groups involved particularly in that sport. However, in any sport it will be remembered that the whole body is used, and circuit training sessions should not over-emphasise one area of the body only.

Planning Strength Schedules

In the past, work with weights was mainly confined to those involved in

The author assisting an Olympic Medallist sprinter during a weight training session.

the sport of weight-lifting, the body-builders who exhibited their improved musculature in competitions (e.g. "Mr. Universe"), and the

"strong men" who toured the world giving demonstrations of their prowess in circuses and at other venues.

Nowadays, weight-**training** has become universally acknowledged as the best means of increasing strength. But present-day sportsmen and sportswomen have not simply adopted the lifting schedules of the weight-lifters and body-builders. The reason for this is obvious; not only are the requirements in each sport different, each **individual's** strength increase requirements differ. That is why coaches and sportsmen should plan **individual** schedules designed to improve strength in particular muscle groups where there is a weakness, as well as schedules to improve the individual's all-round strength.

There are a number of considerations when planning strength schedules:

(a) the sportsman must be

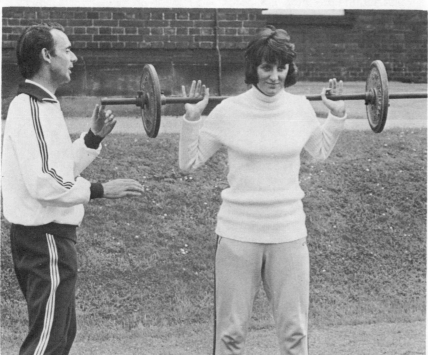

reminded that there is no short cut to improving strength (or skill, or flexibility, or endurance). Improvement comes only as a result of **regular** hard work;

(b) the sportsman's strengths as well as weaknesses should be taken into account;

(c) the schedules should not include too many exercises, concentration on a few is better;

(d) schedules can be split so that sportsmen can work on the arms and upper body on one day, and on the legs and trunk another day;

(e) progress must be **seen** i.e. if as the weeks progress no improvement is made in one particular exercise, it is useful to introduce another exercise instead; and

(f) safety factors must **always** be stressed.

But the main message to all sportsmen and coaches is that participants in all games and sports can benefit from weight-training, and this applies to women as well as men.

Selecting the Exercises

A thorough warm-up in track suit, consisting of some jogging, stretching exercises and fast lifting of a light weight is a cautionary procedure prior to weight training. The exercises that follow will generally depend on the sport for which the participant is training, but a useful method is to include the same two or three exercises on each session for general strength increase, and add two further exercises for the specific needs of the individual.

The exercises should be spaced out so that two or three different arm exercises are not included consecutively. A common method is to have an arm and shoulder exercise, followed by an abdominal exercise, followed by a leg exercise. These would form the "general" strength-ening. The additional specific exercises for, say, footballers (legs) or hammer throwers (arms and back) could follow.

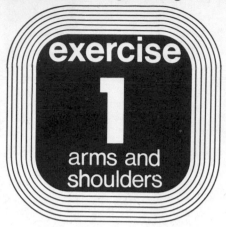

exercise 1 arms and shoulders

MILITARY PRESS

The starting position is with the feet just under the bar, the hands grasp the bar about shoulder width apart, the head is held with the eyes looking up and the breath is held. A top class tennis player here is demonstrating one of the exercises from his schedule.

a

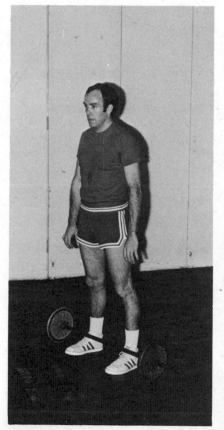

b

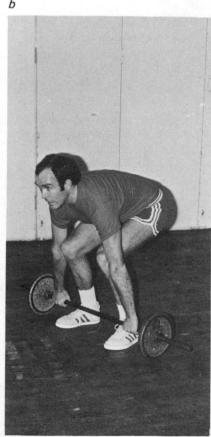

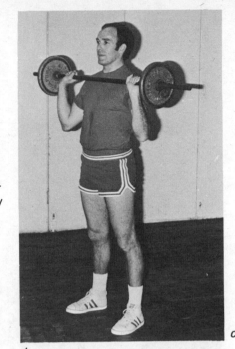

The bar is lifted to the chest by a vigorous pull of the arms and a pushing up of the legs. The back should **not** be jerked into the movement. The wrists are twisted sharply so that the palms are pointing upwards.

c

d

After a slight pause for breath with the bar at the chest, the bar is **pushed** upwards so that the arms are completely straight above the head. The lifter should avoid the tendency to lean back from the waist, for this is the cause of lower back injuries.

e

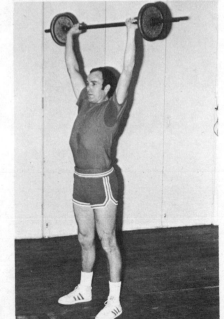

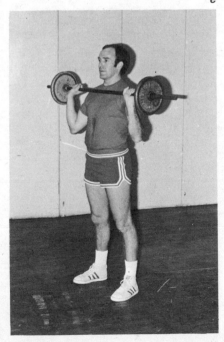

Next the bar is lowered slowly to the chest.

The main purpose of this exercise is to raise the bar from chest into the air a number of times, i.e. a number of "repetitions".

Once the number of required 'repetitions' has been performed, the problem is to return the bar to the floor. This is done with the head up, and **not** stooping with a bent back; the **legs** should be bent and the bar lowered to the floor once more.

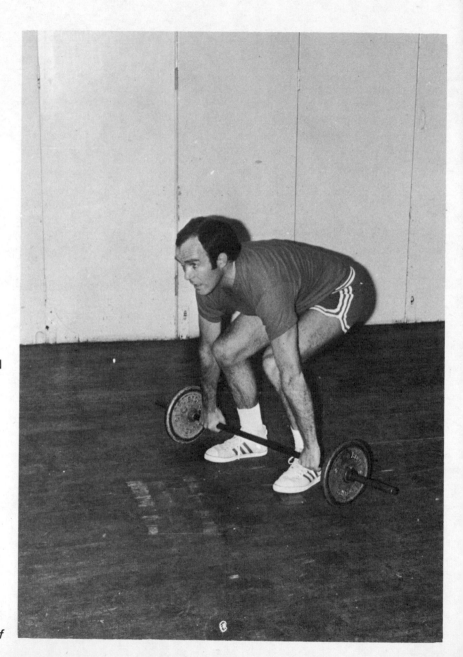

f

The exercise is appropriate for women, though instead of a long bar, two dumbells may be held, with alternate arms pressing a weight above the head. A woman games player demonstrates a valuable arm exercise alternative.

a

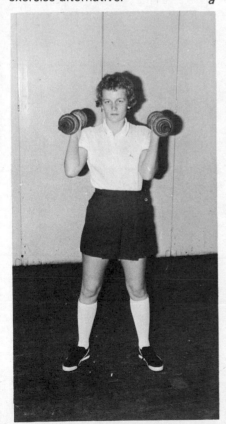

b

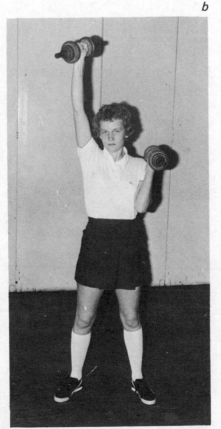

c

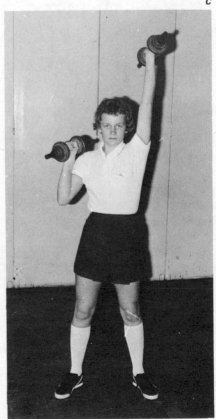

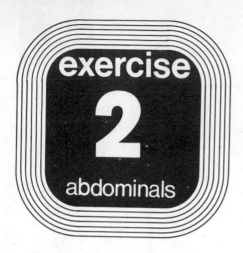

exercise 2 abdominals

TRUNK TWISTS

a

With a weight disc clasped behind the head, the English county cricketer here lies down with his feet anchored by a weight bar, wall bar or a partner holding his ankles. The knees are slightly bent.

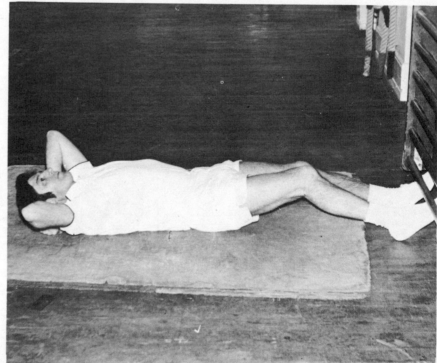

b

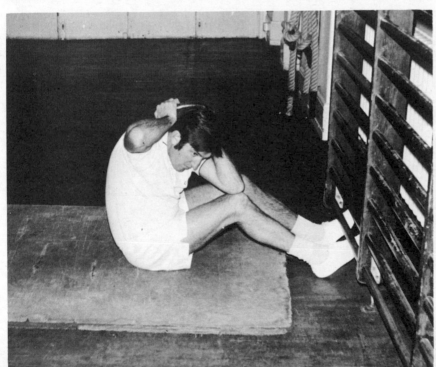

One "repetition" consists of raising
the body so that one elbow touches
the opposite knee (e.g. left elbow to
right knee).

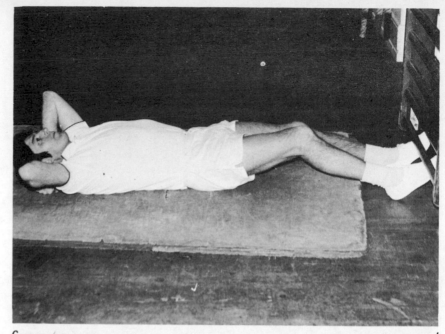

c

d

The person then lies down again, the next repetition would be right elbow to touch left knee etc.

The exercise is safe for women, though of course lighter weights would be used.

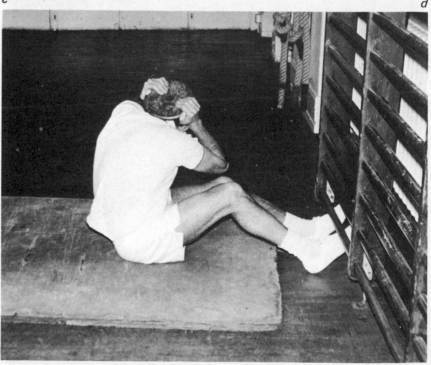

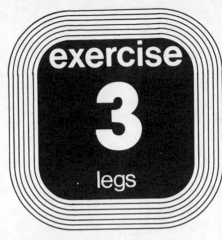

exercise 3
legs

HALF SQUAT

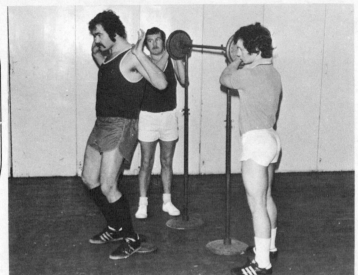

a

b

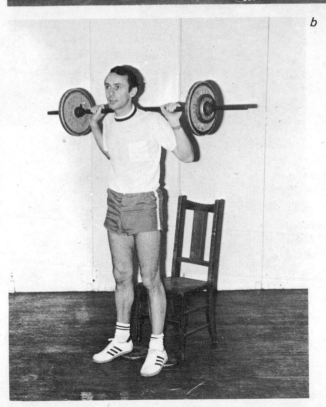

A bar is placed on the shoulders by two fellow sportsmen (if squat stands are not available). The bar is grasped firmly, the head is held up and eyes look sightly upwards. To prevent achilles tendon injuries, the heels are placed about 1 inch off the floor on a block of wood. A chair is placed at the rear of the sportsman, in this instance an Olympic athlete.

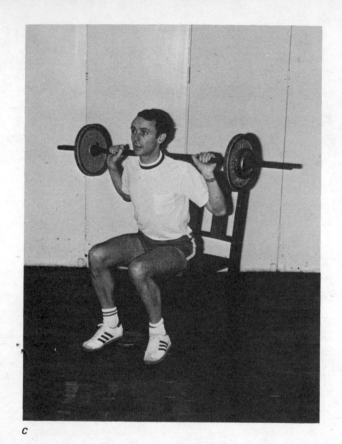

c

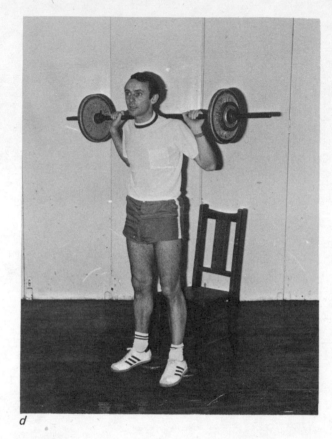

d

The movement is initiated by the legs bending until there is approximately an angle of 90° at the knees (should the athlete go below 90°, injury might result—the chair being there to ensure the athlete does not go lower). The head remains upright.

Some coaches do not like women to use this exercise, though their alternative suggestions often appear not to be leg **strengthening** at all. The main problem seems not that women cannot do the exercise, but that the bar digs more into their necks than it does with men. This pain can be alleviated by wrapping a towel around the bar to pad it.

One repetition is completed when the athlete pushes with his legs (the back should **not** be jerked) until his body is upright again.

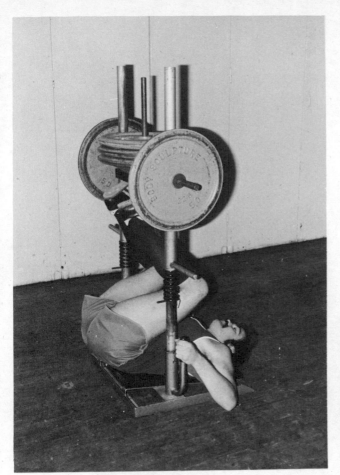

a

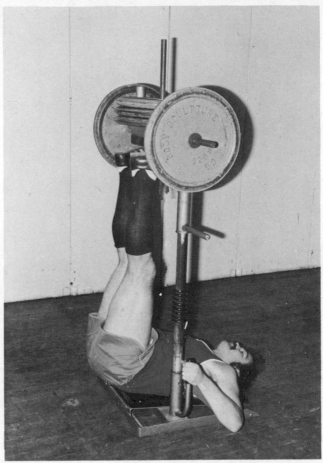

b

Where the facilities include costly machinery, then an alternative to half-squat is a leg press. Here, a top-class rugby player lies down and presses the weight up by using his legs.

Specific Exercises

In addition to the general strengthening, a triple jumper may require to do extra leg work, whereas tennis, squash and badminton players require more forearm and wrist exercises, and crawl swimmers more arm and shoulder exercises. The following are recommended as useful exercises to be added occasionally to the weight training programme.

83

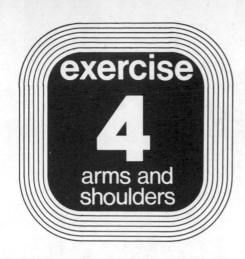

exercise 4
arms and shoulders

BENCH PRESS

The exercise is done with the sportsman, here a top class badminton player, lying on a bench. The bar is passed to him by two friends, or he can lift it from a rack. The bar is held perpendicularly over the chest with arms extended to their fullest.

a

The bar is lowered slowly until it touches the chest.

b

One "repetition" is completed when the bar is explosively returned once more up into the air.

c

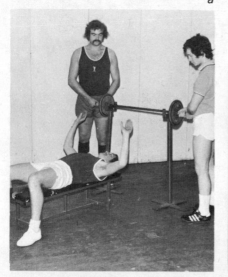

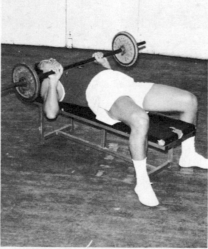

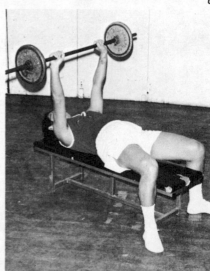

a

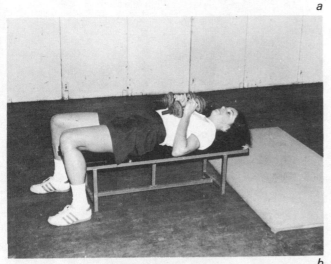

Women may safely carry out this exercise, or use dumbells to punch up alternately. Here an outdoor education enthusiast demonstrates an exercise she uses for toughening up for her sailing, canoeing and rock-climbing activities.

b

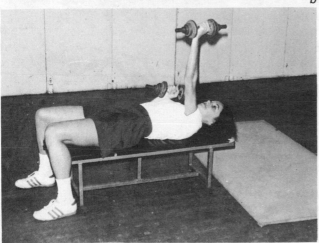

c

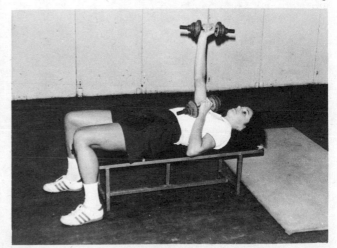

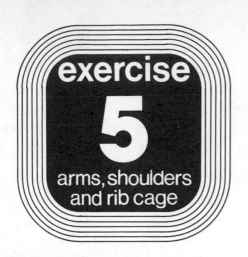

exercise 5
arms, shoulders and rib cage

BENT-ARM PULLOVER

Lying on a bench, the bar is grasped behind the head with hands shoulder width apart. The feet are placed either side of the bench with the flat of the soles and heels on the floor. An Olympic canoeist is seen here demonstrating one of his training schedule exercises.

The effort comes from the arms, kept bent, pulling the bar over the head, then finally pushing the weight to a perpendicular position over the chest.
After a slight pause, the bar is slowly lowered with arms bending, until the weights touch the floor again, one "repetition" having been accomplished.

Women can carry out this exercise safely, though using lighter weights.

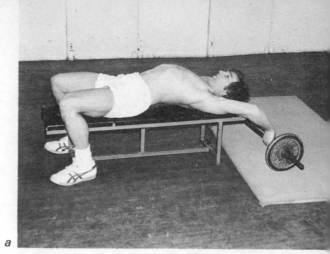

a

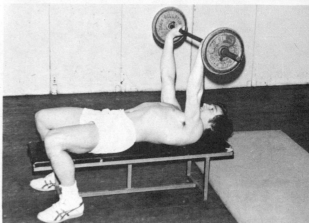

b

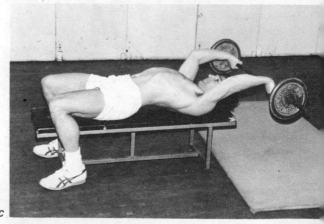

c

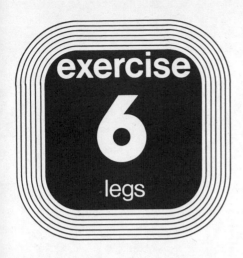

exercise 6 legs

STEP ON BENCH

The bar is held across the shoulders behind the neck. The bench should be of such a height that when one leg is placed on, the knee is at no less an angle than 90°.

a

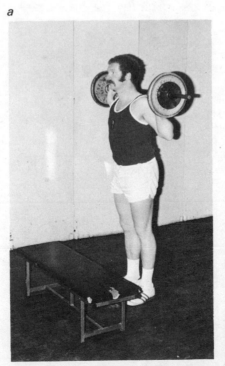

b

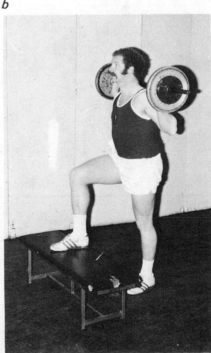

One leg is placed on the bench and the body is raised to a vertical position. Then the sportsman steps down again—one "repetition" has been carried out. The next step up should be done with the other leg, and so on alternately.

Women can carry out this exercise. But they and the men should ensure that it is done at a smooth rhythmic pace, and care must be taken not to bend or twist the trunk during the movement.

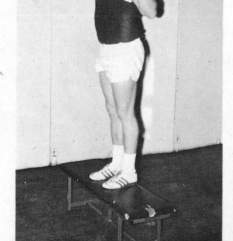

c

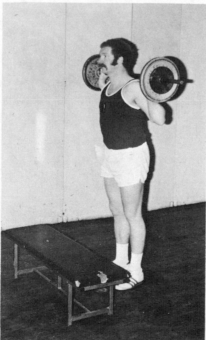

d

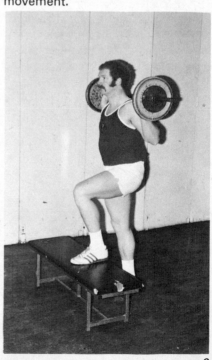

e

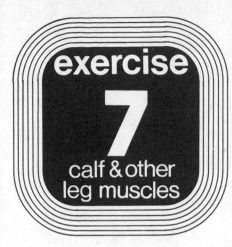

exercise
7
calf & other leg muscles

HEEL RAISE

The weight is held behind the neck, across the shoulders. The toes are placed on a 2 inch block of wood. Here, a rock climber demonstrates an essential activity for those whose sport requires much work using calf muscles.

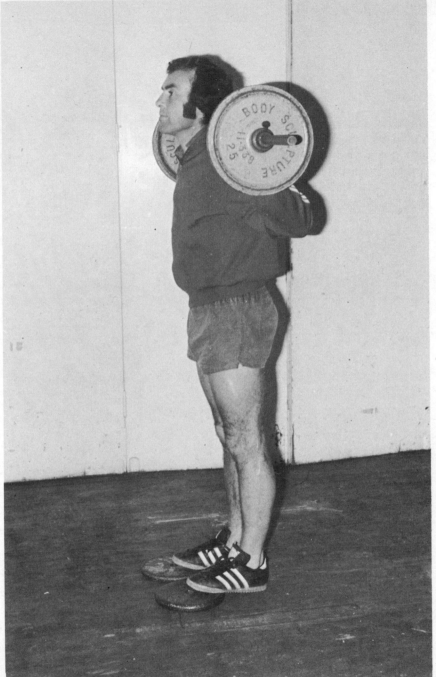

a

89

The body is then raised by the action of the calf muscles raising the heels as high off the floor as possible. A count of about 10 seconds is made, that is the athlete says aloud, "one and two and three and four and five and six and seven and eight and nine and ten".

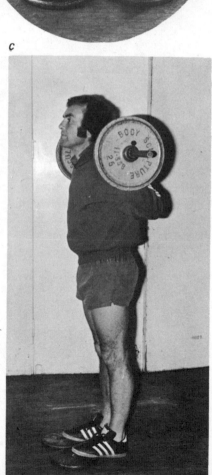

b

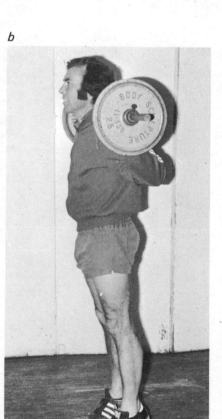

c

Then the heels are lowered to the floor for about ten seconds before the next "repetition".

The exercise can be performed by women, though they (and some men) by experience will alter the time factor.

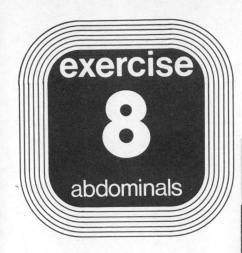

exercise 8
abdominals

LEG RAISE

The starting position is lying on the back. If possible weighted boots can be used, or a medicine ball can be held between the feet. An expert sub-aqua man here uses this abdominal exercise for preparation for his demanding sport.

The feet are then raised slowly until the heels are not quite perpendicular.

After a brief pause with the feet in the air, the legs are lowered to the ground again.

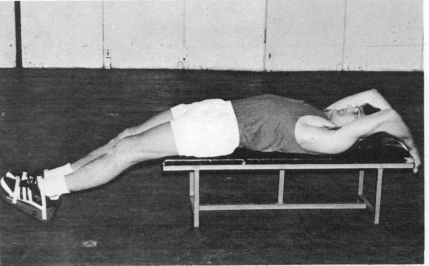

a

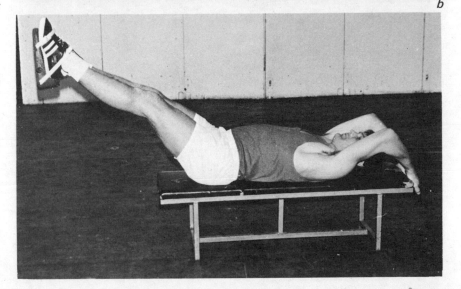

b

The exercise can be performed by women without weights, whereas men can increase the difficulty by adding weight to the boots, slowing down the movement and altering the angle and the pause of the feet in the air, or by doing the exercise on an inclined bench.

a

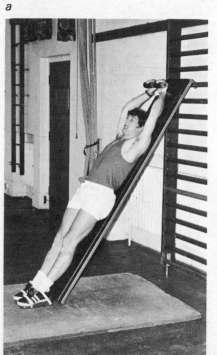

b

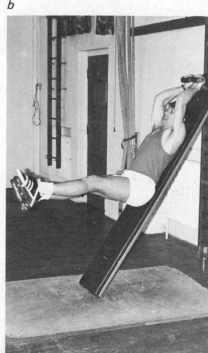

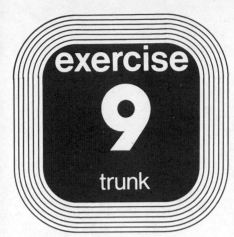

exercise 9
trunk

SIDE BENDS

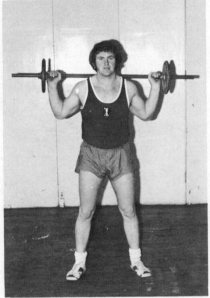

a

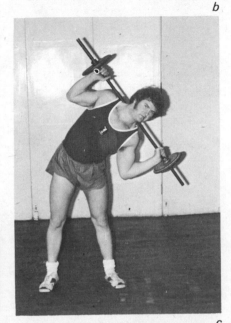

b

Starting position is with the bar held behind the head on the shoulders, **with the collars securely tightened** to prevent the weights sliding off and falling on the floor. Here an athlete (throwing event) demonstrates.

Next the body is bent sideways as far as is possible, but *not* leaning forward *or* backwards.

The body is then returned upright before bending to the other side.

c

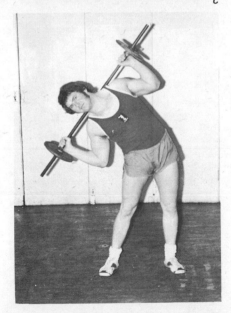

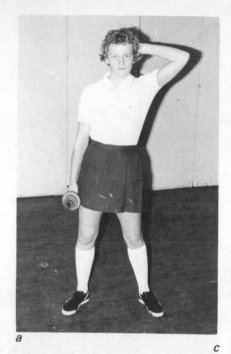

a

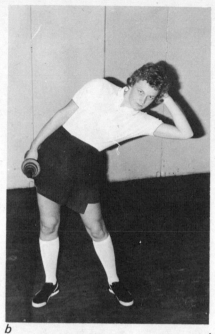

b

c

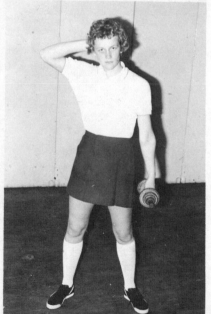

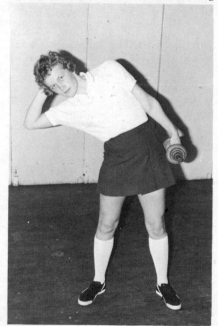

d

Women can do this with lighter weights or simply hold a dumbell in one hand and place other hand behind head, then lean away from the weighted side. Repeat on other side with weight transferred to other hand.

How Much Weight?

When introducing weights or when beginning to include weight-training after a lay-off, e.g. at the beginning of the pre-season training, it is most important that heavy weights are **not** used. In time, the strength will only be increased by use of **heavy** weights, **but** because of the risk of injury, the introduction of new exercises must be through the use of **light** weights for two or three weeks.

The author has found that an excellent method of weight-training is by initially using a light weight (or for women, the bars only with no weights on) and requiring 10 "repetitions" of the exercises done 3 times, with a short rest (say 10 seconds) between each "group" of 10 repetitions. In training schedules, this is usually referred to as 3 sets of 10 repetitions; or:

"3 × 10 with 50 lbs"

means the exercise must be carried out using a total weight (bar, plus collars to secure the weights, plus weight discs) of 50 lbs; the exercises must be done 10 times, then a short rest; then a further 10 times, another short rest, and finally a third series of the 10 exercises.

Once the coach is happy that the man or woman is carrying out the exercise intelligently, effectively and without danger to self and others, he can reduce the number of repetitions to 8 and at the same time increase the weight, i.e. instead of,

3 × 10 with 50 lbs
(total lifted = 1500 lbs)

now

3 × 8 with 65 lbs
(total lifted = 1560 lbs)

It will be observed that the 3 × 10 system is in fact "endurance" activity, and to a certain extent so is the 3 × 8 system. Therefore after a further "probationary period" of two or three sessions, the coach will

again reduce the repetitions and increase the weight, e.g., to

3 × 6 with 90 lbs
(total lifted = 1620 lbs)

The activity is now more a "strengthening" programme and most sportsmen will be adequately strengthened using this system. **More advanced** sportsmen may move to a 3 × 5 or even a 4 × 4 system in some of their exercises, and some will use "multi poundage" or "pyramid" systems. But these systems have to be taught by extremely good coaches, to reliable sportsmen, and with constant supervision. It is generally recommended therefore that men and women use the 3 × 6 or 3 × 5 system.

The weight lifted will depend upon the exercise and the strength and sport of the participant. It is advisable to find out the appropriate weight by experiment, erring on the cautious side to begin with; that is, giving the participant too light a weight. It will be a psychological boost in the early weeks for the participant not to be given weights with which he cannot cope. It is also less likely that he will be injured.

In other words, in the "trunk twist", on the first occasion the athlete will be required to attempt 3 × 10 with a 5 lb disc behind his head. If he manages this comfortably, the next time he can be required to do 3 × 10 with a 7½ lb disc, before reducing to 3 × 8 with 10 lbs. It must be remembered that strength improves only when the participant keeps on increasing the poundage used.

How Often?

The answer to this question would again differ dependent upon the individual's need e.g. a discus thrower might weight-train every day during the winter months when his discus throwing is limited by weather conditions, whereas a distance runner might consider spending even one day's programme solely on weight-training as wasteful.

But a generalisation can be made that about two weight-training sessions of about one hour per week seems to be appropriate for most games players, and during other sessions there would be the emphasis on skill and endurance. Some individual sports participants, e.g. track and field athletes might require three sessions especially during their off-season.

The decision about the frequency depends upon a number of factors. If a games coach prefers to have all of his players together most of the time, he might only wish to have one or two half sessions on weights i.e. one day after a brief weight session, they would be required to practise games skills. Another coach may not wish to devote **lengthy** periods to weights, so he would perhaps require his players to work on different muscle groups each day e.g. warm-up followed by arm strengthening weights then skill session; next day, warm-up followed by adbdominal strengthening weights then skill session; next day, warm-up followed by leg strengthening session then skills, etc.

Weight sessions can be lengthy if the changing of the weights on bars etc. are carried out by one man. It is useful therefore to train in groups of two or three, so that while one is exercising the other two can be helping him to put the weight on his back and be preparing the next weights to be used. Training with others is also a safety measure, can be more enjoyable, and is more motivating.

Some Example Schedules

Male Triple Jumper

Day 1
Warm-up

Military Press	3 × 6 with 60 lbs (aiming eventually to use $\frac{3}{4}$ of his body weight)
Trunk Twist	3 × 6 with 15 lbs behind head
Half Squat	3 × 6 with 120 lbs (aiming eventually to use twice his body weight)
Bench Press	3 × 6 with 70 lbs (aiming eventually to use twice his body weight)
Heel Raise	3 × 6 with 120 lbs (aiming ventually to use twice his body weight)

At Least Two Days Later
Warm-up
Military Press   As before
Trunk Twist   As before
Half Squat   As before
Leg Raise   3 × 6 with weighted boots
Step on bench   3 × 6 with 120 lbs (aiming eventually to use twice body weight)

Female Games Player

Day 1
Warm-up
Alternate Dumb-bell punch   3 × 6 with 10 lbs
Trunk Twist   3 × 6 with 5 lbs
Half Squat   3 × 6 with 50 lbs
Side Bends   3 × 6 with 10 lbs dumb-bells
Bench Press   3 × 6 with 10 lbs dumb-bells

At Least Two Days Later;
Warm-up
Alternate Dumb-bells   As before
Trunk Twist   As before
Half Squat   As before
Bent-arm pullover   3 × 6 with 15 lbs
Heel Raise   3 × 6 with 50 lbs

Other "Strengthening Work"

With no weight-training facilities, some coaches and sportsmen will need to stretch their inventive resources to try to obtain a similar effect in training to that which weight training gives.

The author, when training at a club that could not afford weights, acquired some large tins (cans or drums) which measured about 18 inches high and about 12 inches square at the end. These were filled with concrete and allowed to set with a 6 foot length of metal about 2 inches in diameter placed in the middle. These became useful means of half-squatting. Smaller empty jam tins (or cans) were similarly filled with concrete so that a number of different weights were available. Other methods include using a partner's weight (e.g. on the back) for instance in half-squatting. Or

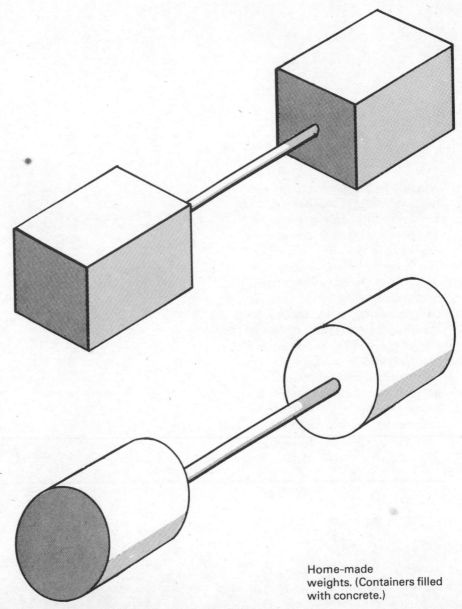

Home-made weights. (Containers filled with concrete.)

hanging by the arms from a beam, raising the legs to touch the beam to the left and the right of the arms as an abdominal strengthening exercises.

The important consideration, however, is that the above are only substitutes, and although expensive weight-training machines are *not* essential, coaches and sportsmen should gradually aim to acquire 6 foot long weight bars, 15 inch bars, various size discs and collars, so that as soon as is possible a more accurate weight programme can be devised and implemented.

The Importance of the Psychological Factor

".. . exercises have definite physiological and psychological values."

Major (1939)

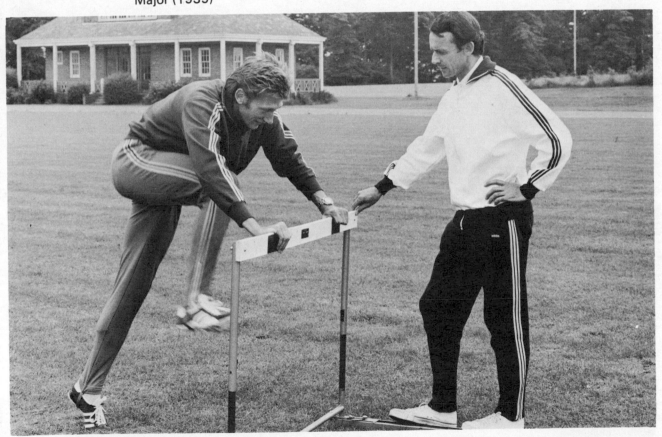

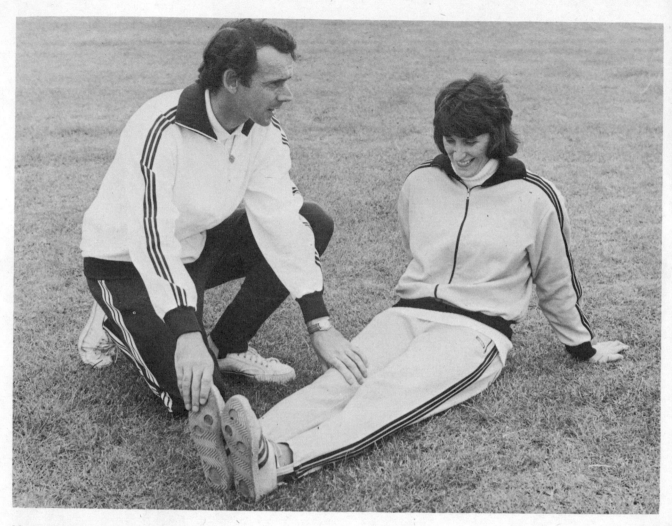

Many successful sportsmen and women prefer not to depend on old-fashioned beliefs. They tend to exchange training hints and discuss the "pros" and "cons" of new-found knowledge.

Here the author discusses coaching points with an Olympic 400 metre hurdle medallist and a woman Olympic sprinter medallist.

Tradition

Many coaches, trainers and sportsmen have beliefs about the value of particular training routines or "big-match" preparation that are based more on misplaced faith or superstition rather than on proven worth. Such idiosyncrasies include the need to swallow a raw egg whipped in sherry on the day of a competition, the need to eat a large steak for lunch on the day of a competition, and the wearing of the same suit of clothes, shirt, socks, tie etc., that were worn on the last day the team won!

Unfortunately, as the years progress, with the sportsmen being required to retain a particular apparently worthless routine, the difficulty to shake the faith in these practices increases. That is to say some psychological benefit **is** obtained by some players from them, because they obtain comfort from the routines that are traditional in their club, or that their coaches require. The problem arises when due to illness, minor accident, lapse of memory, etc. the routine is broken. At these times the sportsmen may then perform **badly** as a result of the breaking of a worthless routine. For example, when a manager or coach leaves a team, there has to be a period of adjustment to the idiosyncrasies of a new leader, and during this time not only individuals', but the whole team's performance may suffer. As in previous Chapters, what needs to be emphasised is that individuals should **not** all be expected to adhere to the **same** psychological treatment either in training or on competition days.

It is therefore profitable to consider some of the psychological factors that affect a person's performance in competition and training, and to illustrate how a rational attitude should more often be adopted towards them

Practice

Many sportsmen, sportswomen, coaches and trainers believe that "practice makes perfect". But they fail to realise that many of their practices are bad techniques, therefore what in fact they are perfecting are bad faults! In order that the result of practice or training is **improved** performance, the practices **must** be related to the actual performance required on the day of the competition. For instance:

(a) games teams should train in similar coloured shirts to those they wear on the day of the match, for they need to be able to react quickly to pass the ball to one of their own team by reacting to a blur of a familiar colour;

(b) if they are to play occasionally in inclement weather, sportsmen should practise in inclement weather, and not go into the gymnasium on wet days to train;

(c) if their game consists of playing against opposition, they should train against opposition, so that not only is their accuracy of, say, passing the ball subjected to distraction, but they should be tackled and knocked to the floor too if that is what happens in the game;

(d) it may be necessary to train for only phases of a game rather than attempt to provide an identical full match situation. If so, these phase practices must also be realistic;

(e) in individual sports, there is also a need for opposition to be provided in training. A sprinter could set a not-so-good athlete ten metres ahead of himelf as opposition, rather than merely completing a number of sprints alone;

(f) where possible, distractions such as crowd noises need to be included in training sessions. For instance relay-runners could practise baton-exchanges while fellow athletes shout and clap during the passing of the baton. Whatever practises or training schedules are designed, they should always be purposeful, realistic situations related to the actual game or performance, and not isolated sessions based on whims or personal preferences.

Feelings

How one is "feeling" has an effect upon one's performance in training and during competition. Family problems can adversely affect performances, therefore coaches should make it their duty to ensure that they know when family difficulties arise which might be on the mind of the sportsmen or sportswomen. **Also,** coaches should be aware of any effect that training or competitions are having on the sportsman's family life.

Another situation in which a sportsman's feelings can affect his performance is when he is surrounded in training or competitions by players better than himself. An example is the games team where nearly all are "stars" or famous players; the individuals who do not belong to this category could well be made to feel inferior, and when one begins to **feel** inferior one performs in an inferior fashion. Coaches should help to boost the morale of those who feel in such a way about their own ability in relation to their colleagues', or in the case of individuals, those who feel that their next opponent is someone who is very superior.

There are simple ways of ensuring that teams or individuals feel differently about their own ability. A new set of attractive shirts in which to play, a new badge to wear, a new travelling uniform, new track suits, staying at good hotels before competitions, and general "special" treatment to make the sportsmen feel "special". The only cure for some, however, is for them to transfer to a team at a lower level, or for individuals to take on a lower standard of opponent.

Anxiety

Feelings of inferiority can of course create anxiety. But there are other situations not normally recognised which can cause over-anxious feelings in sportsmen. It is necessary for sportsmen to feel slightly anxious because in such situations they will perform well when their adrenalin is pumping into their systems. But a too anxious state renders sportspeople ineffectual. A common cause of over-anxiety is bullying by coaches, trainers, parents etc. Everyone does not react favourably to shouts of abuse. The fact is that **some** men and women **do** perform better when insults are hurled at them, but others are affected **adversely** by over-enthusiastic, bawling coaches. Unfortunately, in many sporting situations, it is erroneously considered "good" coaching when the coaching instructions are loud. In fact many of the best coaches perform very effective duties unobtrusively. **Good** coaches know which are the lazy sportsmen who need to be chased and which are those sensitive ones who require the quieter approach.

Encouragement

One of the most effective methods of ensuring progress in coaching is the use of encouragement or praise. As with children, sportsmen often react favourably to praise and it acts as an incentive to further effort. The encouragement in some sports will be in the form of financial bonuses, or the nomination as "man of the match", or a special commendation. In most circumstances, the friendly congratulation will suffice.

Progress

For sports people, knowing **how** one is progressing is vitally important. Previous chapters have referred to test scores and objective methods of indicating how the "fitness" is improving. These spur on an athlete if friendly rivalry is engendered. However, there is a danger that at some point in time, a sportsman's actual progress is not so good, and this often coincides with his being low in morale. The dilemma for the coach is whether or not to allow the sportsman to be tested at these times, for the poor result will deflate his ego, whereas telling him that he is not up to the standard to take the test could have a similar result. The author has found one solution in such circumstances. I have permitted the man or woman to take the test, but deliberately have allowed extra time without their knowing it, so that a false indication has been the result. Additionally, I have added up the weights incorrectly so that the athlete thought he was lifting more than in fact he was. This method is of course a moral question of whether coaches should ever deliberately deceive those in their care. Some would say that if the consequence is of advantage to the sportsmen, then it could be justified.

"To distil human strength into speed and skill and to elevate mankind's mind above the weakness of reward and recognition . . . that is the sole purpose of sport."

BALJIT S. GREWAL (India)

Personality

Finally, when one looks around at the physical make-up of those involved in the various sports, one will perceive different colour of hair, different colour of eyes, different heights, different weights, and generally different types of build. What **also** has to be remembered is that in psychological make-up, all of these sportsmen and women are quite different.

In earlier chapters, a plea was made for different schedules or programmes of physical conditioning to be devised for individuals. It must also be stressed that individuals also need **individual** treatment psychologically. A different method of explaining the practice, a different amount of time at the practice, perhaps a modification of the practice, or possibly an elimination of the practice altogether might be required within one small group of sportsmen. On the day of competition, a different treatment will be needed among a group. Some will need to be constantly in conversation, some will need to be constantly alone, some will actually be sick, some will be apprehensive, some will need to be bullied.

Sportsmen and sportswomen themselves must also learn these facts, and remember that what is good for one successful person in their sport may not necessarily be good for them. The success of any individual in sport depends largely on his discovering (or his coach's discovering) how **he** is best prepared in order to compete at his highest level of ability. Faith in the methods of conditioning must be present, and a tendency to "change horses in mid-stream" must be avoided. Furthermore in training and competition the purpose of what one is doing should always be remembered.

HOW FIT ARE *YOU*?

Everyone, including non-athletes, secretly would like to be able to discover how fit they are. Sportsmen speak glibly about being almost 100% fit, and usually base this statement more on pride than on measured performance. When I am asked for a quick indication of someone's fitness, I show them the following figures, and tell them to compare themselves with the scores I have taken of various sporting groups:

Comparative Fitness
(Muscular Endurance Tests)

Average Scores in Sixty Seconds

	Burpees	Press-ups	Trunk Twists	Squat Jumps	Totals
Physical Education Students	34	37	38	57	166
Top English Soccer Players	33	30	36	55	154
Top English Rugby Players	28	32	32	54	146
English County Cricketers	28	23	28	43	122
English National Athletes	Score highest on all of these tests				

Having glanced at the above, most people draw conclusions such as: "physical education students are fitter than other groups" and "soccer players have stronger legs than rugby players" and "cricketers tend not to be fit" whereas "international athletes are the fittest of all". Next they compare their own scores with the list, then they tend to make excuses for their own poor scores. I simply allow them to test themselves and worry at their lack of fitness or delight in their scores compared with the table above. Then I insist that they answer a number of questions:

1. What does the above table really imply?
2. How does one differentiate between a prop forward's fitness and that of a wing-threequarter in the rugby scores above?
3. Would a goalkeeper be expected to be equated with a mid-field player in soccer?
4. Would an international athlete's fitness enable him to withstand the bruising in games playing?

In other words, most testing should be of an individual's progress and he should not compare himself with other people who have different types of bodies from himself, and different talents. Simple tests as shown above are useful guides to intelligent coaches, but conclusions from them should be drawn with caution.

Testing should be done; testing acts as a motivation; but tests can also be misleading.

BIBLIOGRAPHY

Karpovich, P. V. (1965). *Physiology of Muscular Activity.* W. B. Saunders & Co.

Major, E. (1939). *Medicine-ball Exercises and Games.* University of London.

Morgan, R. E. and Adamson, G. T. (1957). *Circuit Training.* G. Bell & Sons.

Pickering, R. (1968). *Strength Training.* A.A.A. London.